Praise for *The 4-Week Ultimate Body Detox Plan:*
A Program for Greater Energy, Health, and Vitality

"Michelle shares her compelling story of healing with wisdom and compassion as she gently guides you through this exceptional book. Read her book carefully and put into practice her simple, straightforward, commonsense principles, and you will be glad you did for the rest of your long and healthy life."

—HARVEY DIAMOND, #1 *NEW YORK TIMES* BESTSELLING COAUTHOR OF *FIT FOR LIFE*

"Michelle's detox plan is an elegant, gentle, yet life-saving methodology, well-conceived through personal experience and thoroughly grounded in research. I heartily recommend it."

—MEG JORDAN, PhD, RN, EDITOR-IN-CHIEF OF *AMERICAN FITNESS*

"After the first week or so, you settle into a routine, get more adventurous in the kitchen, and start to really enjoy feeling good about the healthy choices being made. My *4-Week Ultimate Body Detox Plan* results: Lost—5 pounds; Gained—a much healthier attitude to food; Upside—My clothes fit better. I feel better. I'm eating better food and having way more fun in the kitchen. Insomnia is a thing of the past. Walking has become a regular part of my life. Downside—none."

—ROBIN SUMMERFIELD, CONTRIBUTING EDITOR, *CALGARY HERALD*

WEEKEND WONDER DETOX

Also by Michelle Schoffro Cook:

60 Seconds to Slim:
Balance Your Body Chemistry to Burn Fat Fast!

The Ultimate pH Solution: Balance Your Body
Chemistry to Prevent Disease and Lose Weight

The 4-Week Ultimate Body Detox Plan:
A Program for Greater Energy, Health, and Vitality

The Phytozyme Cure: Treat or Reverse More Than 30
Serious Health Conditions with Powerful Plant Nutrients

The Life Force Diet: 3 Weeks to Supercharge
Your Health and Stay Slim with Enzyme-Rich Foods

The Brain Wash: A Powerful, All-Natural Program to
Protect Your Brain Against Alzheimer's, Chronic Fatigue
Syndrome, Depression, Parkinson's, and Other Diseases

WEEKEND WONDER DETOX

Quick Cleanses to
Strengthen Your Body and
Enhance Your Beauty

Michelle Schoffro Cook,
MS, PhD, RNCP, ROHP

Da Capo
LIFE
LONG
A Member of the Perseus Books Group

Designed by Trish Wilkinson
Set in 11.5 point Goudy Oldstyle Std by the Perseus Books Group

Cataloging-in-Publication data for this book is available from the Library of Congress.

First Da Capo Press edition 2014
ISBN: 978-0-7382-1736-9 (paperback)
ISBN: 978-0-7382-1737-6 (e-book)

Published by Da Capo Press
A Member of the Perseus Books Group
www.dacapopress.com

Note: The information in this book is true and complete to the best of our knowledge. This book is intended only as an informative guide for those wishing to know more about health issues. In no way is this book intended to replace, countermand, or conflict with the advice given to you by your own physician. The ultimate decision concerning care should be made between you and your doctor. We strongly recommend you follow his or her advice. Information in this book is general and is offered with no guarantees on the part of the authors or Da Capo Press. The authors and publisher disclaim all liability in connection with the use of this book.

Da Capo Press books are available at special discounts for bulk purchases in the US by corporations, institutions, and other organizations. For more information, please contact the Special Markets Department at the Perseus Books Group, 2300 Chestnut Street, Suite 200, Philadelphia, PA, 19103, or call (800) 810-4145, ext. 5000, or e-mail special.markets@perseusbooks.com.

10 9 8 7 6 5 4 3 2 1

This book is dedicated to the love of my life,
my husband, Curtis.
Never before have two loved more.

CONTENTS

1   Why You Need to Detox   1

2   Getting Ready to Detox   31

3   The Love Your Liver Weekend   65

4   The Lymphomania Weekend   95

5   The Kidney Flush Weekend   117

6   The Colon Cleanse Weekend   145

7   The Skin Rejuvenation Weekend   173

8   The Fat Blast Weekend   201

9   Keeping the Detox Spirit Alive
    After the Weekend's Over   235

10 Recipes   239

    About the Author   277

    Acknowledgments   279

    Resources   281

    Notes   285

    Index   291

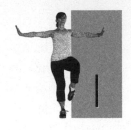

WHY YOU
NEED TO DETOX

Detox has never been more popular. That's because it works. And it helps us get our diet and lifestyle back on track after any excesses we've experienced or to help us reach our health goals quickly and efficiently. Some people turn to detoxification because they binged on too many carbs. Others seek out a cleanse to prepare for a wedding or reunion. Still others want to shed pounds or improve their skin. Whatever the reasons for detoxifying, *Weekend Wonder Detox* can help. Whatever the reasons for cleansing, few people realize that we're inundated with toxins in our everyday life that can interfere with our ability to experience optimal weight and health. For millennia our bodies relied on built-in mechanisms to keep cells, organs, and internal systems working in the face of pathogens, exposures to naturally occurring poisons, wounds and infections, and an assortment of other, potentially dangerous forms of toxicity found in the natural world. Although the human body evolved to detoxify and protect itself naturally against these things, with varying degrees of success, the introduction of thousands of synthetic chemicals, including food additives and pharmaceutical medicine, has created a toxic burden with which the body is easily overwhelmed.

Human beings today are carrying a greater toxic load than at any other time in history. It is manifesting itself in sky-high rates of "environmental" and "lifestyle" diseases like diabetes, obesity, cardiovascular and respiratory disease, and cancers. Whether it is household cleaners, air fresheners, personal care products, or medicine, the toxic chemicals they contain may pose challenges to even the finest-tuned detoxification systems. This truth extends to our food supply as well, as food and beverage companies continue to find ways to incorporate chemicals and synthetic ingredients into the products the public consumes, frequently without their knowledge. The distinction between food processing and chemical industries as well as the pharmaceutical industry is becoming increasingly blurred, at the expense of your health.

The good news is that there are a lot of things you can do to protect yourself from toxins. In reality, detox just makes good sense if you want your body to perform at its best. Think of it this way: How do you take care of your computer? Do you protect it from shocks and extremes of temperature; load it with recognized and reputable software, including programs to protect it from viruses; keep the keyboard and screen clean from foreign debris and dirt; and regularly perform maintenance, cleaning, and upgrading to ensure it stays working at optimum levels? Most of us spend more time on the proper functioning of our computers than we do on our own health.

Even with this level of care, many people replace their computers every few years or less. But we don't have this luxury with our bodies, so we need to maintain and protect them by reducing their exposure to harmful substances and activities. Despite the prevalence of toxins in our body, detoxing is not as difficult as you might think—and the rewards are amazing. More energy and vitality, improved weight management, improved moods, clearer skin and thicker hair, and an improved ability to fight off harmful viruses, bacteria, fungi, and other assorted bugs and disease.

Still not convinced? Still think your liver, kidneys, bowels, or sweat glands will take care of any toxins that find their way into your body? Think again. Because our bodies were not designed to ingest and filter out the myriad chemicals we're exposed to daily, they get stored in our tissues, usually in fat. They can build up to a point that they create a toxic load that overwhelms the body, creating all kinds of symptoms linked to various forms of disease.

These toxins are a 24/7 reality. Few of us hear about the health effects of PCBs, DDT, BPA, and other toxic chemicals. When it comes to toxins lurking in your food, beverages, water, home, and personal care products, what you don't know *is* hurting you.

Did you know that over eighty thousand chemicals find their way into the environment? And where do they end up? In your food, water, air, and, ultimately, your body! Consider this shocking reality about cancer: the International Agency for Research on Cancer has concluded that *80 percent* of all cancer is attributable to environmental influences, including exposure to carcinogenic chemicals. These are not only chemicals from the smokestacks and effluent pipes of giant industrial corporations; these are also chemicals you will pick up by the dozens in your regular grocery order at the local supermarket or the fast-food line-ups in your neighborhood.

We'll get into detail about the toxins below; in this Age of Toxins you can no longer afford to stand by and hope your body can cope with the onslaught of harmful, sometimes carcinogenic, toxic chemicals it comes in contact with. You *need* to give your body's detoxification systems a boost. It all begins with one three-day weekend. Of course, you can repeat the weekend as often as you like or do one weekend each month or different weekends periodically to give your body a serious boost. The choice is yours. The Weekend Wonder Detox is flexible and targeted to your individual needs. Forget the one-size-fits-all detox that doesn't consider your unique needs. These detox weekends have been designed with flexibility in mind—you can target specific areas and customize the plan.

THE POWER OF
THE WEEKEND WONDER DETOX

Detoxification programs don't have to be arduous, lengthy, costly, and minimally effective. That's the old-school detoxification regime. I know this from experience, both professionally and personally. I am a doctor of traditional natural medicine, clinical nutritionist, herbal medicine practitioner, and an orthomolecular health specialist (I use nutrition as medicine to help people overcome illnesses). I've been a natural health professional for over two decades. I've also tried just about every detox program available. Some worked, some didn't work, and some were dangerous. I developed the Weekend Wonder Detox as a way to transform what I call "deprivation detoxification" into a spa weekend that goes beyond the "puff and buff" approach I see so often.

I asked myself, "Why can't transforming your body, looks, and life feel fun and exciting and still be effective?" and "What could be easier or more practical than a weekend detox?" The Weekend Wonder Detox is my answer to these questions. The weekend detoxes create a spalike feeling rather than a feeling of deprivation that most people experience on other detox regimes. The detoxes you'll find here are easy and straightforward: three days filled with delicious toxin-busting superfoods, gentle herbal remedies, and balancing natural therapies that will have you feeling great in only one weekend.

You'll leave lethargy behind, shed excess weight, and watch skin outbreaks disappear. Get to the bottom of uncomfortable health issues: toxic buildup that clogs healthy organ function. Every herb and nutrient used in the *Weekend Wonder Detox* is scientifically proven to protect, boost, rebuild, or strengthen the organs for which I selected them. I selected them because they work and are backed by sound research.

Although our bodies are designed to handle some toxins, they can rarely handle them in unlimited quantities over prolonged periods of time. Giving your body some support through foods, nutrients, herbs, exercises, and therapies will help ensure your body operates at peak function rather than just getting by.

Of course, you can eliminate toxins as little or as often as you'd like. You'll discover several weekend cleansing options enabling you to focus on the detoxification organs or systems in your body that need the most help. Just select the weekend that works for you, and pick the Weekend Wonder Detox that fits your needs. Don't worry—I have developed a short quiz in Chapter 2 to help you determine where to target your efforts: the liver, lymphatic system, kidneys, intestines, skin, or fat deposits. Once you've discovered the organs or systems that need a tune-up you can target them to send toxins packing. You can focus on only one weekend, repeat it periodically if you'd like, or you can work your way through multiple cleanses or even do them all over several weekends.

Choose from the Love Your Liver Weekend, the Lymphomania Weekend, the Kidney Flush Weekend, the Colon Cleanse Weekend, the Skin Rejuvenation Weekend, and the Fat Blast Weekend. No matter how busy your schedule or stressful your life, you can benefit from Weekend Wonder Detoxes. And, of course, it's not necessary to use every therapy recommended in each chapter. In addition to the full dietary suggestions, simply choose the therapies that most appeal to you—the more the better. You'll also incorporate the power of aromatherapy, energy medicine, acupressure, meditation, and ancient healing exercises like qigong and yoga postures that target key areas of your body.

You'll quickly discover as you continue to read that *Weekend Wonder Detox* is not a "boot camp" approach to health. I don't believe in breaking people's spirits or treating them like garbage as they embark on a healing journey. I believe in a holistic, mind-body-spirit approach to detoxification, including foods, juices, herbs, and exercises to strengthen the body. *Weekend Wonder Detox* offers meditation, breathing exercises, acupressure, energy medicine techniques, aromatherapy, qigong, yoga, and other natural therapies that will balance your mind and spirit as well as your body.

My goal is to empower you to take charge of your life by delivering health and healing information in a practical, do-it-yourself format. These detoxes are easy to follow and easy to use. Forget the lengthy, cumbersome detoxes that are impossible for most people to follow. I bet you'll love it for a weekend . . . and love it for a lifetime. You can pull out the *Weekend Wonder Detox* again and again whenever your body needs a boost or your organs need a "tune-up."

Before we dive right into the detoxes, let's just take a look at some of the toxic substances in the common foods, beauty, personal care, and household products you use. The things I am about to tell you may shock you or make you feel a bit overwhelmed. That is not my intention. It is important to be informed to make the best choices for your health and the health of your loved ones. Please remember that the best way to eliminate toxins from your body is to stop exposing yourself to them. Say "no" to companies that fill their products with harmful toxins because they are cheap or lengthen the shelf life of their products. Your health is worth more than their profits. Also remember that we are going to explore ways to eliminate or reduce toxins to which you have already been exposed.

OUR MODERN FOOD DILEMMA

Since the start of the Industrial Age a century and a half ago the quality of our food supply has been on the decline. It has been subjected to degradation that would shock most people. Even some of the healthiest foods are no longer healthy choices.

Our food supply now contains everything from plastic residues, pesticides, synthetic colors, artificial sweeteners, excessive amounts of natural sweeteners or so-called natural sweeteners that are chemically altered, industrially altered fats (trans fats), rancid oils, and genetically modified organisms (GMOs). Some food barely resembles food any longer and more aptly reflects the industrialization of our food supply that has been occurring over the last century or so. Let's explore some of these dietary shortcomings.

Plastic Food and Other Things You Shouldn't Put in Your Mouth

If you wrap your food in heat-resistant plastic before boiling or cooking, there's a good chance that the toxic chemicals in plastic are leaching into your food. Guess what: whoever eats this food has just been subjected to the many toxic ingredients found in plastic, which just leached into their food, contrary to what the chefs may tell you.

Plastic finds its way into food through plastic containers, microwaving food in plastic wrap or containers, drinking water from plastic water bottles, and storing food in plastic bags.

One of the most toxic ingredients in plastic is a hormone disruptor called bisphenol-A (BPA). Even in miniscule amounts—scientists are discovering that sometimes smaller amounts are worse than large amounts with hormone disruptors!—it can wreak havoc on our delicate hormonal balance and lead to a whole host of health problems or weight gain. Even if you're trying to watch your weight, plastics may be thwarting your best weight loss efforts.

A new study from Harvard School of Public Health, published in the journal *Environmental Health*, found that commonly found toxins in plastics arc linked to both general and abdominal obesity. Harvard scientists found that the higher the levels of BPA in urine, the more likely a person was to be obese and to experience abdominal obesity.[1]

As a result of studies like the Harvard one, BPA, PCBs (polychlorinated biphenyls), and phthalates are increasingly being referred to as "obesogens." That's because they are being linked to weight gain and obesity. If you want to lose weight, getting the chemicals out of your diet, home, and body are critical. I'll discuss phthalates a bit later in this chapter, but here is some important information about PCBs.

The ABCs of PCBs

Farmed fish, particularly salmon, is a source of a toxic group of chemicals known as polychlorinated biphenyls, or PCBs. PCBs are increasingly showing up in other parts of the food supply, including in chicken, beef, pork, eggs, and even milk. PCBs are proven carcinogens. They were banned in the seventies in both the United States and Canada, and possibly elsewhere, but they still show up in our food supply because they are so persistent in the environment.

Color Me Toxic

The next time you're at a child's birthday party notice the beautiful array of cakes, cookies, and cupcakes, all showcasing a rainbow assortment of artificial colors. Although they may make these sweets look appetizing to children, these synthetic ingredients often take the place of nutrition in foods. For example, fruit juice that contains colors is typically devoid of any fruit, making it artificially colored sugar water. Worse than that, many food colors are linked to hyperactivity disorders and even cancer.

Although the names of the dyes are meaningless to most people (yellow 5 or tartrazine, which is derived from coal tar, and blue 2 or indigotine, for example), their effects are not. These toxins are commonly found in concentrated fruit juices, condiments, and some cheeses, to name a few sources. A study in *The Lancet*, a reputable, mainstream medical journal, brought wide attention to this health concern. Blue dye numbers 1 and 2 have been linked with cancer in animal tests, and red dye number 3 caused thyroid tumors in rats. Green dye number 3 was linked to bladder cancer, and yellow dye number 6 was linked to tumors of the kidneys and adrenal glands. These colors are readily used in most processed, prepared, and packaged foods.

Natural Sweeteners and Other Urban Myths

Just because a sweetener is originally derived from a food source doesn't make it a healthy option in your diet. There are many food-derived sweeteners that are anything but healthy. And even the healthier options are not healthy when eaten in the quantity with which most people eat them. A small amount of honey is fine for most people, but it still causes rapid blood sugar fluctuations that are in turn linked to mood swings, energy crashes, and weight gain.

There isn't sufficient room to discuss the pros and cons of every sweetener here, but I would like to discuss some of the problems linked with sugar and artificial sweeteners. In the next chapter I'll make suggestions regarding natural sweeteners to use on the *Weekend Wonder Detox.*

Sickly Sweet Sugar

Sugar is one of the most addictive substances on the planet. Volumes of books can be written on the widespread damage sugar does to the body, and it has as much to do with the amount we eat as it does with the toxic nature of the stuff (I can't in good conscience call it food). Individual human consumption of sugar in most parts of the world has increased more than twenty-five times over the last century. Five generations ago a five-pound bag of sugar was a full year's supply. Now, most people eat that much in two weeks!

Sugar is found in virtually all processed, packaged, and prepared foods. It is even found in salt sold by some food manufacturers. Remember, we are not talking about naturally occurring sugars in fruit, vegetables, grains, and legumes. We get more than enough sugar in our diets by eating these foods without adding additional sugars through processing or preparation. Industrial sugar processing has brought this sweet killer to more and more people over the last century, increasing a host of diseases and disorders that have reached epidemic proportions.

The connection between sugar consumption, weight gain, and increasing rates of obesity should be clear to just about every adult by now. It has been known for decades. It's one of the "bad carbs" in the good carbs–bad carbs argument. The same can be said about sugar consumption and diabetes. But it is sugar's link to so many other prevalent health problems like heart disease, high blood pressure, high cholesterol, and premature aging that escapes our attention. What about allergies, hormonal problems, excessive

mood swings, and depression? Sugar consumption has been impli-
cated in all of these health problems.

It is important to take charge of the food choices we make.
Read the labels on packages, but don't be fooled if the word sugar
isn't listed. Sugar goes by many names, most of which end in the
letters "ose," like fructose, lactose, maltose, and dextrose. You will
make a giant leap in detoxifying your body by eliminating these
sugars from your grocery list and your diet. It is more difficult if
you like to eat out; however, it is safe to assume that fast-food
chains, family-friendly restaurants, and even most upscale dining
establishments will be heavy-handed with the sweet, white toxin.

The Other Fattening "Natural" Sweetener

Most people assume that a sweetener that is purportedly derived
from a "natural" source must be a healthy option, but, in our modern era of industrial processes applied to every aspect of life, including food processing, "natural" really doesn't guarantee superiority
when it comes to food. This is particularly true because most regu-
lators allow the claim "natural" to appear on almost anything.

High-fructose corn syrup goes by the names corn syrup, corn
sweetener, or fructose, all of which sound harmless enough, but
they are anything but. This harmful sweetener has been linked to
obesity, high blood pressure, and many other health issues.

Corn syrup is the sugar extracted from corn. When isolated it is
not and never has been healthy, but as corn is now almost entirely
genetically modified, it is even worse for us. High-fructose corn
syrup is high in fructose—hence the name—and it quickly con-
verts to fat in your body. Actually, when some scientists study obesity in experimental animals, they frequently give them HFCS to
make them obese. What's more is that this food additive is found
in most packaged, prepared, and fast foods. It not only causes most
people to store fat; it also interferes with appetite control and hormones linked to metabolism.

Food manufacturers use this sweetener because it is cheap and
makes us eat more and crave more. And it shows in our bottom
lines. Just eliminating this sweetener for good is enough to cause

most people to lose weight and regulate high blood pressure. According to a University of Colorado study published in the *Journal of the American Society of Nephrology*, researchers found that even people who eat a healthy, low-sodium diet may be at risk of high blood pressure due to the consumption of HFCS as an additive, as it was shown to increase blood pressure by up to 32 percent.[2] HFCS increase also causes inflammation in the bloodstream, which constricts blood vessel walls, thereby increasing the risk of heart attack and stroke.

HFCS is found in most processed, packaged, and prepared foods and condiments but is especially common in soda and foods labeled "low fat" or "nonfat." Here are some surprising sources of HFCS:

- Baby food
- Cereal (even so-called healthy cereals or cereals intended for children)
- Condiments
- Crackers
- Granola and granola bars
- Salad dressing
- Yogurt

You'll want to start reading labels to make sure you are avoiding high-fructose corn syrup, corn syrup, corn sweetener, or fructose.

A Sweetener by Any Other Name Still Stinks

Sugar-free foods and beverages are usually full of artificial sweeteners concocted in a laboratory, including aspartame (now called NeoTame or AminoSweet), saccharin (Sweet'N Low), or sucralose (Splenda), and these artificial sweeteners are even worse than their sugary counterparts.

The Toxin That's Had a Makeover

Thanks to slick marketers, the artificial sweetener Aspartame now goes by the ever-so-sweet-sounding name of "AminoSweet."

Surely a substance with such a lovely name is safe for use? Let's consider aspartame, er, AminoSweet's history to answer that question.

First developed in 1974, by 1980 an FDA Board of Inquiry voted unanimously AGAINST approving aspartame for human consumption, but by 1983 the FDA commissioner Arthur Hull Hayes Jr. overruled the vote. Only one year after the approval an FDA task force learned that some of the original data showcasing aspartame's safety had been falsified to hide results showing that animals fed aspartame had developed seizures and brain tumors; however, the FDA maintained—and still maintains—its approval of this product.

By 1991 the National Institutes of Health catalogued 167 adverse effects linked to aspartame use. In 1992 the US Air Force issued a warning to pilots not to fly after ingesting aspartame. And by 1994 the US Department of Health and Human Services had linked the artificial sweetener aspartame to the risk of 88 symptoms of toxicity.

According to Lynne Melcombe, author of *Health Hazards of White Sugar*, research links aspartame to the following health conditions:

- Anxiety attacks
- Appetite problems, such as binge eating and sugar cravings
- Birth defects
- Blindness and vision problems, such as blurred vision, bright flashes, and tunnel vision
- Brain tumors
- Chest pain
- Depression and emotional problems
- Dizziness and vertigo
- Edema
- Epilepsy and seizures
- Fatigue
- Headaches and migraines

- Hearing loss and tinnitus
- Heart palpitations and arrhythmia
- Hyperactivity; insomnia
- Joint pain
- Learning disabilities
- Memory loss
- Menstrual irregularities and PMS (premenstrual syndrome)
- Muscle cramps
- Nausea
- Numbness of extremities
- Psychiatric disorders
- Reproductive problems
- Skin lesions
- Slurred speech
- Uterine tumors

Research even links aspartame to death. Aspartame's effects can be mistaken for Alzheimer's disease, Amyotrophic lateral sclerosis (Lou Gehrig's disease), chronic fatigue syndrome, epilepsy, Epstein-Barr virus, Huntington's chorea, hypothyroidism, Lyme disease, Ménière's disease, multiple sclerosis, and post-polio syndrome.

According to Randall Fitzgerald, author of *The Hundred-Year Lie*, some of the cancers linked to aspartame include brain, liver, lung, kidney, and lymphoreticular cancer.

Aspartame is found in many diet products, including soft drinks, as well as a wide variety of prepared foods. Shockingly, it is also found in some multivitamins, supplements, and pharmaceutical drugs.

And, here's a shocker: according to the authors of the book *Hard to Swallow*, when a diet drink containing aspartame is stored at 85 degrees Fahrenheit for a week or longer, "There is no aspartame left in the soft drinks, just the components it breaks down into, like formaldehyde, formic acid, and diketopiperazine, a chemical which can cause brain tumours. All of these substances are known to be toxic to humans."

Saccharin—Long-Term Use
Does Not Equal Safety

Saccharin was created when researchers were looking for coal tar derivatives for commercialization. It goes by many names, including Sweet'N Low, Sweet Twin, and Necta Sweet. But no matter the names, it is still a coal tar derivative.

When it was first researched it was shown to cause bladder tumors in rats but was allowed to stay in the marketplace due to consumer demand, provided it came with a warning label that it may be harmful to health. However, experts still define saccharin as a "probable carcinogen,"[3] and it causes breathing difficulties, headaches, skin eruptions, and diarrhea in some people.

Splenda Isn't So Splendid

Splenda—sucralose—is widely touted as a natural sweetener, but it's not. It was created in a laboratory by altering sugar molecules in a way that could not appear in nature. The artificial sweetener was hardly tested before being launched on an unsuspecting public as a supposedly healthy alternative to sugar. According to research by Dr. Joseph Mercola, the FDA conducted two human studies on sucralose prior to its approval of Splenda and to determine whether it should be allowed in our food. The longest study lasted only four days and only examined sucralose for its effects on tooth decay, not any other health effects. Additionally, when sucralose was tested to determine its absorption in the body, only eight men were studied.

It is not the natural stuff that manufacturers claim it is. It is a chlorinated artificial sweetener designed in a laboratory and created in manufacturing facilities. It may start as a sugar molecule, but the similarities end there. Three chlorine molecules are added to each sugar molecule, which, according to Dr. Mercola, means it "has been altered to the point that it's actually closer to DDT and Agent Orange than sugar." Here is a list of symptoms and conditions that have been linked with sucralose consumption:

- Allergic reactions such as facial swelling, swelling of the eyelids, tongue, throat, or lips
- Allergic skin reactions such as itching, swelling, redness, weeping, crusting, rashes, eruptions, or hives
- Anxiety
- Blood sugar increases
- Blurred vision
- Breathing problems, including shortness of breath, coughing, chest tightness, and wheezing
- Depression
- Dizziness
- Gastrointestinal problems, including diarrhea, vomiting, nausea, bloating, gas, or pain
- Headaches
- Heart palpitations
- Itchy, swollen, watery, or bloodshot eyes
- Joint pains
- Mental fog
- Migraines
- Seizures
- Sinus congestion, runny nose, or sneezing
- Weight gain

Why is this allowed in our food? Splenda's manufacturers tell consumers that its products don't get digested and, therefore, absorbed by the body. Well, that's true, but it's not a positive spin on this toxic product. Splenda is so resistant to breaking down that it is even finding its way into our water supply, which means that many people are unsuspectingly drinking sucralose every day in their water. Researchers took samples from nineteen American drinking water treatment plants that provide drinking water for over 28 million people. They found sucralose in

- the source water of fifteen out of nineteen drinking water treatment plants tested;

- the finished water of thirteen out of seventeen water plants; and
- eight out of twelve water distribution systems.

Once it finds its way into the water supply, sucralose is likely to find its way into your drinking water. So how is your body supposed to deal with this toxic compound? It can't. As for its presence in your water supply, I'll discuss ways to deal with water filtration and purification later in this book. But for now I want to be sure you're aware that sucralose is not fit for consumption.

Fat That's Not Fit to Eat

Most people consume a large amount of harmful fats in their diet, either in the form of excessive amounts of saturated fats (in small amounts it isn't harmful, but most people eat way too much of this fat) and trans fats, which are extremely toxic no matter how much you eat. Saturated fat is found primarily in animal products such as meat, poultry, and dairy products.

We also eat high amounts of rancid and overheated oils in processed, packaged, and prepared foods, fried foods, cooking oils, margarine, shortening, and lard. Although healthy fats are found in fresh, raw fruit and vegetables, nuts, seeds, and grains as well as in oils derived from these ingredients, oils in our diet are typically rancid largely because they are old, have been processed incorrectly, have been exposed to light or oxygen for too long, or have been excessively heated. The oils found in grains, nuts, and seeds are heated to over 500 degrees during processing. That high level of heat alters the biochemical structure of most oils, turning them from potentially healthy foods into rancid and harmful toxins.

Additionally, during storage the oils used in many packaged foods are also exposed to excessive amounts of light and oxygen, which can destroy their beneficial properties. This means that once-beneficial fats cause inflammation when consumed.

But overheated and rancid oils are not the only fats to be concerned about. Trans fats have been the topic of much public discussion over the last decade, so you're likely familiar with them. Trans fats have been linked with countless diseases, causing them to become banned in places like New York City.

Trans fats are a recent construct and would not have appeared in our ancestors' diets even a century ago. Yet we are eating them to the tune of five pounds of trans fats annually. In an attempt to process them, the liver is put under a tremendous amount of strain. Our intestines cannot break down or absorb these fats, so they attempt to neutralize them, causing the loss of essential minerals like calcium and potassium.

Stanford-trained research scientist Dr. J. Robert Hatherill found that diets containing trans fats make brain cell membranes excessively permeable, which allows viruses greater access to the brain, disrupts brain signals, causes brain cells to become dysfunctional, and promotes cognitive decline.

Trans fats do not just affect the brain though; they are damaging to the whole body. They cause inflammation throughout the body. Inflammation, in turn, has been linked to cancer, heart disease, arthritis, diabetes, and many other illnesses.

Hydrogenated and trans fats are found in margarine, shortening, or products made with them. That includes baked goods, cookies, pies, buns. Switching from cookies, crackers, pies, French fries, and snack foods that contain trans fats to ones made with healthier oils will go a long way toward improving your brain and mental health.

ABCs of MSG

Monosodium glutamate, or MSG as it is more commonly known, is linked to many serious health conditions, including hormonal imbalances, weight gain, brain damage, obesity, headaches, and more—you may be shocked to learn how prevalent it is. MSG is almost always found in processed, prepared, and packaged foods.

But here are some lesser-known food sources of this harmful chemical:

Soup—Most soups, even most homemade soup, contains MSG, even if the cook swears it doesn't. That's because most soup bases, commercial stocks, and bouillon powder and cubes contain MSG.

Spice Mixtures—Love that Cajun seasoning, TexMex rub, or other spice mixture? Most spice mixtures contain MSG, frequently as autolyzed yeast or yeast extract.

Infant Formula—As terrible as it sounds, some infant formula actually contains MSG in one of its myriad disguises.

Soy "Meat" Products—Many of the vegetarian burgers, hot dogs, sausages, or other meat alternatives contain textured vegetable protein (TVP), hydrolyzed vegetable protein, or hydrolyzed plant protein, all of which usually contain MSG.

Baby Food—Shocking as it is, manufacturers of baby food often include glutamate, one of MSG's many guises, as a flavor "enhancer."

Bottled Sauces—Just gotta have your Thai, Teriyaki, or Jamaican Jerk sauce? Well, most bottled sauces contain MSG.

Salad Dressings—The salad dressing you're choosing could be negating any of the health benefits of eating salad if you choose a bottled dressing that contains MSG. Bottled salad dressings may contain "natural flavor," "spices," or "seasoning," all of which can legally contain MSG.

Salad Croutons—Most croutons are flavored with bouillon, soup base, or "natural" or artificial flavors that contain MSG.

Protein Powder—Many of the protein powders used for weight loss or muscle building, even those sold in health food stores, can contain MSG, usually as hydrolyzed protein or hydrolyzed soy protein.

Vaccines—Many vaccines contain MSG or glutamate. The chickenpox as well as the measles, mumps, and rubella (M-M-R) vaccines are two common examples.

According to board-certified neurosurgeon Russell Blaylock, MD, author of *Excitotoxins: The Taste That Kills*, here are some of the many names for this harmful toxin so you know what to look for on food labels:

Additives that always contain MSG:

- Monosodium glutamate (that's the full name for MSG)
- Hydrolyzed vegetable protein
- Hydrolyzed protein
- Hydrolyzed plant protein
- Plant protein extract
- Sodium caseinate
- Calcium caseinate
- Yeast extract
- Textured protein
- Autolyzed yeast
- Hydrolyzed oat flour

Additives that frequently contain MSG:

- Malt extract
- Malt flavoring
- Bouillon
- Broth
- Stock
- Flavoring
- Natural flavoring
- Natural beef or chicken flavoring
- Seasoning
- Spices

Additives that sometimes contain MSG

- Carrageenan
- Enzymes

- Soy protein concentrate
- Soy protein isolate
- Whey protein isolate

Next time you're buying packaged foods be sure to take this list with you to avoid harmful neurotoxins that could be affecting your health.

Frankenfoods and More Freaks of Un-Nature

What if I told you that there are corporations unleashing bacteria shells that contain viruses that spread pesticides instead of infection in our food supply? I know it sounds like something out of a disturbing and far-fetched science fiction movie. When people say "reality is stranger than fiction" I think they might be talking about genetically modified foods.

The brainchild of various corporations, with Monsanto being the most well known and holding the largest market share of genetically modified organisms (GMOs), these frankenfoods threaten our food supply and environment on a scale that has never been seen before.

Consider the production of potatoes that need to be transported in a hazardous waste container because every cell contains pesticides. Or, worse than that, that these cells continue creating pesticides once you've eaten them and they are inside your body. Governments around the world never insisted on extensive safety testing of genetically modified ingredients before allowing them to be unleashed on unsuspecting people. The US FDA even publicly stated, "The FDA has not found it necessary to conduct comprehensive scientific reviews of foods derived from bioengineered plant . . . consistent with its 1992 policy."[4]

Yet independent researchers found nineteen studies linking genetically modified foods with disease in animal studies.[5] They found that a diet that includes GMOs significantly affects the blood and urine biochemistry as well as organ weights. But the

FDA didn't think it was necessary to test them prior to allowing them to be widely available to the American public. And now the Grocery Manufacturers of America estimates that 75 percent of all processed foods in America contain at least one genetically modified ingredient.

The result of the nineteen studies indicates a wide range of health problems linked to GM food consumption. They include intestinal damage, allergies, liver or pancreatic problems, testicular cellular changes, tumors, and even death in the experimental animals.

The important message that comes out of the studies is the importance of eating organic and avoiding genetically modified foods at any cost. We simply don't know enough about the long-term effects of eating food that has been artificially tampered with using the genes from other species. GM foods should never have been "grandfathered through" as "generally recognized as safe" (GRAS) by the FDA, Health Canada, and other organizations when there was insufficient research on their safety.

There are five main foods that have been heavily genetically modified. Although there are many more genetically modified foods and food ingredients than that, these five are the most widespread. They, unfortunately, hide in most packaged, prepared, and processed foods, so eating fresh foods or organic foods will help you steer clear of the worst culprits, which include:

- **Corn**—GM corn is found in most foods now, usually as high-fructose corn syrup, corn syrup, corn starch, corn flour, cornmeal, corn oil, dextrose, fructose, glucose, and "modified food starch."
- **Soy**—Soy is largely genetically altered too. The way to avoid GM soy is to be sure you choose "Certified USDA Organic" or "Certified Organic" soy from a reputable certifying agency. That includes foods like soy milk, soybeans, soy flour, soy oil, tofu, miso, tempeh, soy sauce, and other soy-based foods. It also includes food or supplements containing

lecithin, protein isolate, vegetable oil, vegetarian protein, and isoflavones.

- **Canola**—Most canola is not what it used to be. It is now grown from genetically modified seeds. It is found in canola oil, vegetable oil, and rapeseed oil. If you're baking, choose coconut oil or organic extra-virgin olive oil instead.

- **Cotton**—Okay, I know you're thinking, "Cotton! But I don't eat cotton!" And that may be true, but, if any of the processed, packaged, or prepared foods you're eating contain cottonseed oil, then be aware it is likely derived from GM cotton.

- **Sugar**—Unless your sugar-containing foods are labeled "100% cane sugar," "100% organic sugar," or "evaporated cane sugar," it is likely derived from sugar beets. And those beets were likely genetically modified. Choose coconut sugar or coconut sap instead. Not only does it taste great, but it is also a healthier option anyway. One teaspoon contains only three grams of sugar instead of the four grams of white sugar. That may not seem like a big deal, but when you consider that the average person eats over 150 pounds of sugar a year, just switching to coconut sugar would reduce that intake by a whopping 37.5 pounds a year!

The genetic modification of our food supply could be the topic of an entire book, and there are many good ones devoted to this topic. Check out the resources section at the back of this book for more information.

THE UGLY SIDE OF BEAUTY PRODUCTS

Our quest for beauty and attractiveness may be damaging our health and the health of the planet. Many personal care products contain toxic ingredients that we need to avoid, yet they are commonly found in most commercial products, from toothpaste to shampoo, to makeup and hair styling products. Here are some of the most common ingredients and the products in which they are typically found, along with the health problems to which they are linked:

Methyl, propyl, butyl, and ethyl parabens—Used to extend the shelf life of products, they are highly toxic, carcinogenic, and cause skin conditions.

Synthetic colors—As with food colors, these colors go by names like FD&C or D&C followed by a number. They are known to cause cancer. Even toothpaste and toothbrushes contain these harmful ingredients. Yes, that toothbrush with the colored bristles that supposedly tells you when to throw out your toothbrush is a problem. The dye is readily absorbed through the mucus membranes in your mouth into your bloodstream. Choose products devoid of colors or ones that obtain their color from natural earth minerals and pigments.

Petrolatum—Mineral oil and jelly that promotes sun damage and leads to dry skin and chapping as well as skin conditions. Products containing petrolatum usually claim to alleviate the very conditions they create. It is found in petroleum jelly products and even in baby oil.

Sodium laurel sulphates—Used in shampoo, body wash, and soap to cause lathering, it also causes skin conditions, hair loss, eye irritations, dandruff, and allergic reactions. Avoid products that contain this ingredient even if it is supposedly sourced from coconut.

Imidazolidinyl urea and diazolidinyl urea (Germall II and Germall 115)—Commonly used preservatives in many personal care products and cosmetics and cause skin conditions. The latter releases cancer-causing formaldehyde when it is above 100 degrees Fahrenheit.

PVP/VA copolymer—A petrochemical used in hairspray, perm solutions, and many cosmetics. The particles may stay in the lungs, causing respiratory concerns.

Stearalkonium chloride—Used in hair conditioners and skin creams, it is a highly toxic ingredient developed by the fabric industry originally as a fabric softener. (Yes, that means fabric softeners are toxic too.)

Fragrance—Any of over four hundred ingredients, mostly derived from petrochemicals, "fragrance" causes hyperpigmentation of skin, headaches, asthma, joint pains, muscle pain, fatigue, swollen lymph nodes, raised blood pressure, dizziness, rashes, skin irritation, and coughing, to name a few. Choose products that contain only essential oils (not "fragrance oils") if you want a scent. Better yet, make your own perfume blend with essential oils. For more on this, see Resources.

Dioxin—A known carcinogen, dioxin is used in many feminine hygiene products such as tampons and pads. Dioxins absorb through the skin and are linked to immune disorders, endometriosis, and cancer of the reproductive system. Choose natural feminine products devoid of dioxin from your health food store.

Fluoride—Stay clear of toothpaste that contains fluoride. The average person is getting excessive amounts of fluoride from water. Fluoride does *not* protect teeth, and excessive amounts of fluoride are linked to cancer.

Coal tar—Found in most hair dyes, coal tar is linked to numerous types of cancer, including non-Hodgkin's lymphoma. Choose natural hair colors or hennas if you must dye your hair.

Lead—A heavy metal linked to brain disease and many other illnesses, lead is commonly found in many cosmetics, particularly lipstick.

You may be thinking that I am telling you to avoid personal care rituals and hygiene, but I'm not. There are many great natural products free of toxic ingredients at your local health food store. There are natural shampoos, conditioners, soaps, moisturizers, perfumes, hair dyes, toothpaste, toothbrushes, feminine hygiene products, and many others. If you don't like one brand, don't assume all natural products are ineffective. Many work far better than their chemical counterparts. You'll be glad you made the effort . . . and so will Mother Earth.

It's important to choose natural alternatives to the toxin-laden beauty products most companies are selling. But remember that there are few regulations governing the use of the word "natural" on personal care products. I've been approached by representatives at many companies who have told me that their products are "totally natural." Yet when I check out the ingredient list they are not natural at all. Read ingredient lists—and take this book with you if you need a reminder of the possible toxins to watch out for. But remember that this book doesn't contain an exhaustive list— there are thousands of toxins being used in our products. Also remember that, if there is no ingredient list, it's fair to assume the manufacturer is hiding something. Make a trip to your natural food store to find healthier options. It is important, however, to realize that not everything sold at your local health food store is healthy or free of toxins.

CLEANING UP TOXINS IN HOUSEHOLD, WORKPLACE, AND CLASSROOM CLEANING PRODUCTS

The Environmental Working Group (EWG), a nonprofit environmental organization, commissioned a study of the twenty-one most commonly used cleaning products in California schools— although it is highly likely that these are the same products used elsewhere in America and around the world. They used a leading laboratory specializing in air pollution released by cleaning products. Their findings are alarming.

They identified 457 air contaminants released by the twenty-one cleaning products. Comet Disinfectant Powder Cleanser emitted the most, at 146 contaminants released. The fewest contaminants detected were found in Glance NA, a certified green glass and general-purpose cleaner. It emitted only one contaminant.

Twenty-four of the chemicals in the cleaning products have well-established links to asthma, cancer, and other serious health concerns. Twelve of the chemicals are on the State of California's Proposition 65 list of chemicals that are linked to birth defects, reproductive toxicity, and cancer. Ten products contained at least one of the cancer or developmentally damaging and birth defect–causing chemicals on the California list, including Alpha HP, Citrus-Scrub, Comet, Febreze Air Effects, Goof Off, Pine-Sol, Pioneer Super Cleaner, Shineline Seal, Simple Green, and Waxie Green.

Cleaning products that weren't certified green released an average of thirty-eight different contaminants *each*—almost five times higher than certified green ones that released an average of eight contaminants each. Certified green cleaning products contained one-quarter of the chemicals linked to asthma and cancer than the noncertified cleaning products. The laboratory determined that cleaning classrooms—their focus was on classrooms, but the results apply to homes and workplaces too—with certified green products releases less than one-sixth of the air pollution of conventional cleaners.

Here are some of the worst offenders found in cleaning products, along with the health risks of each:

- **Benzene**—linked to cancer and male reproductive system toxicity
- **Chloroform**—causes cancer and developmental toxicity
- **Dibutyl phthalate**—damages male and female reproductive systems
- **Formaldehyde**—causes cancer

What's also shocking is that manufacturers are legally required to disclose only a handful of ingredients in cleaning products.

The Air We Breathe

So-called air fresheners are among the worst culprits when it comes to toxins. They contain many toxic ingredients, but one in particular, phthalates, has been linked with abnormally developed male genitalia, poor semen quality, low testosterone levels, and other reproductive issues. Phthalates are only *one* of the nasty ingredients found in air fresheners, sanitizers, and deodorizers.

An *MSN* article found that being exposed to so-called air fresheners as little as once a week can increase your odds of developing asthma by as much as 71 percent and can contribute to an increase in pulmonary diseases. A 2006 study found that people with high blood levels of the chemical 1.4 dichlorobenze, which is commonly found in popular air fresheners, were more likely to experience a decline in lung function.

Here are some of the ingredients found in the popular metered air fresheners—you know, the ones that are battery operated and pump out mists of supposed sanitizers several times an hour:

Acetone—This is a blood, heart, gastrointestinal, liver, kidney, skin, respiratory, brain, and nervous system toxin. So, in other words, it can damage just about any part of your body and have a wide range of adverse effects.

Butane and isobutane—Yes, we're talking about lighter fluid—in air fresheners! It is a serious toxin to the brain and nervous system.

Liquified petroleum gas and petroleum distillate—It is fairly obvious why we wouldn't want to add this to our air supply. I've been half-jokingly telling my clients for years that air fresheners contain the byproducts of gasoline that the oil industry can't put into vehicles. It looks like it may not be far from the truth.

Propane—Okay, so we all know that we shouldn't barbecue in a closed environment or indoors, so does it make sense to put propane in air fresheners for indoor use? I don't think so. Propane is a cardiovascular and blood toxin as well as a liver, kidney, respiratory, skin, and nervous system toxin known to be extremely dangerous.

Perfume—This single ingredient contains up to four hundred different toxic ingredients, 95 percent of which are derived from petroleum products and are linked to a whole list of serious health conditions ranging from headaches and dizziness to depression and behavioral changes.

Benzene—This is known to cause leukemia in humans.

Formaldehyde—This has been linked to cancers of the upper airways.

And the bottled, canned, plug-in, and other types of air fresheners and sanitizers contain most of the same toxic ingredients. Ironically, these products come with warning labels that state, "Deliberately . . . inhaling the vapor of the contents may be harmful or fatal" or "Avoid inhaling spray mist or vapor." Yet we've been duped into thinking that we need these products to protect us from harmful bacteria or viruses, even though there is no evidence that they actually disinfect the air at all. However, the evidence is mounting that these chemical products harm us—sometimes irreparably.

Obviously the biggest issue is that these ingredients really shouldn't be allowed in products that will be sprayed into the air, inhaled, or absorbed directly into the bloodstream through skin contact. But there are other issues like duping the public into thinking that these products are somehow cleaning the air and eliminating odors—they simply mask them.

TOXINS ARE ALMOST EVERYWHERE . . . SO NOW WHAT?

I know it is a bit overwhelming to learn that so many of the foods, beauty, and household products we've come to rely on are full of toxic ingredients, but, when it comes to toxins, ignorance is not bliss. Being informed helps you make better choices for you and your family so that you will not experience the health ramifications linked to so many toxins.

Now that you understand the number and volume of toxins around us, I think you'll probably agree that it is important to give your detoxification organs a boost. They need it now more than ever. In the next chapter you'll discover how to eat a toxin-free diet and take a quiz to help you focus your attention on the organ or organs most in need of attention.

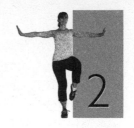

GETTING READY
TO DETOX

Our bodies are exposed to many toxins, as you've just discovered. But that doesn't mean we need to sit idly by and worry about the damage they cause. We can significantly reduce the number of toxins in our life by making simple switches to healthier, more natural, toxin-free products. We can also empower ourselves by strengthening our body's detoxification channels so that they are better capable of handling these toxins.

Before we get started on the essentials of the Weekend Wonder Detox, I encourage you to take the following quiz to determine which organ or organ system is most in need of support so you can choose the best weekend detox for you. Then read the frequently asked questions (FAQs) section below, as it will answer the most common questions I am asked, including, "How often should I detox?" "Which weekend detox should I try first?" and "Is it safe to detox for more than a weekend?"

Let's get started with the quiz. Check each of the symptoms you *currently* experience. If you are not currently experiencing them but had them at another time in your life, do not check the symptom or condition. Do not check diseases or disorders for which you have not received a physician's diagnosis. For example, do not check chronic fatigue syndrome if a doctor never diagnosed you with it, even if you have long-term fatigue; there are more symptoms than lengthy fatigue that are required to obtain such a diagnosis. Be honest with yourself while completing the quiz. Remember: the goal of the quiz is to ensure that you select the best detox for your body right now. The only way to ensure that is to be honest about your health as it stands now.

There is no section that pertains to the Fat Blast Weekend. That's because most people know if excess weight is their highest priority. If weight loss or fat loss is your main goal, you can simply bypass the quiz, read the essentials of the Weekend Wonder Detox as outlined later in this chapter, and then go directly to Chapter 8, where you will learn how to target fat in your body through detoxification. I still encourage you to take the quiz below, as it is an excellent opportunity to learn about your body and its needs. You can go directly to the Fat Blast Weekend, but you may discover that your liver could use a boost too. That would give you insights into a possible additional weekend detox you could use.

Grab a pencil and a calculator, and let's find out what part of your body would benefit from a tune-up.

THE WEEKEND WONDER DETOX QUIZ

Section A
- —— abdominal bloating
- —— alcohol intolerance
- —— allergies
- —— arthritis
- —— asthma
- —— bowel infections
- —— "brain fog"
- —— chronic fatigue syndrome (CFS) (diagnosed by a doctor)

— colitis

— Crohn's disease (diagnosed by a doctor)

— depression

— difficulty losing weight

— environmental illness or multiple chemical sensitivities

— fatigue

— fatty liver

— fevers

— fibromyalgia (diagnosed by a doctor)

— fluid retention

— gallbladder disease

— gallstones or gravel

— gastritis

— headaches and migraines

— hepatitis

— high blood pressure

— high cholesterol levels

— hives

— hypoglycemia (unstable blood sugar levels)

— hormone imbalances

— immune system disorders

— indigestion

— irritable bowel syndrome

— mood swings

— overweight or obesity

— poor appetite

— poor digestion

— recurring nausea and/or vomiting with no known cause

— skin conditions (eczema, psoriasis, acne, rosacea)

— slow metabolism

Score 1 point for each symptom/illness checked. Add the total here _____. Now divide this number by 14 and multiply the answer by 100. Write the final number here _____.

Section B

- — abdominal bloating
- — aches and pains
- — bloating or edema of your bodily tissues
- — cellulite
- — chronic fatigue syndrome (diagnosed by a doctor)
- — fatty deposits
- — fibromyalgia (diagnosed by a doctor)
- — lumps or growths on your body
- — lupus
- — multiple sclerosis
- — other chronic immune system disorder
- — overweight or obesity
- — puffiness around the eyes

Score 1 point for each symptom/illness checked. Add the total here _____. Now divide this number by 14 and multiply the answer by 100. Write the final number here _____.

Section C

- — back pain
- — blood in your urine
- — cloudy urine
- — congestive heart failure
- — dark-colored urine
- — difficult, frequent, or painful urination
- — edema or bloating
- — frequent chills, fevers, or nausea
- — high blood pressure
- — kidney or bladder cancer
- — kidney stones
- — puffiness around the eyes

— swollen fingers, ankles, legs, etc.

— urinary tract infections (UTIs)

Score 1 point for each symptom/illness checked. Add the total here _____. Now divide this number by 14 and multiply the answer by 100. Write the final number here _____.

Section D

— abdominal pain or cramping

— acne

— allergies

— anxiety

— any disorder of the digestive tract

— autoimmune disorders (rheumatoid arthritis, lupus, Hashimoto's thyroiditis, etc.)

— back pain (especially lower to midback)

— bad breath

— bloating

— burping

— "brain fog"

— brittle nails or hair

— chronic fatigue syndrome (diagnosed by a doctor)

— coated tongue

— constipation

— diarrhea

— eczema or psoriasis

— fatigue

— fibromyalgia (diagnosed by a doctor)

— flatulence

— food sensitivities

— frequent sore throats

— heartburn

— hemorrhoids

— high cholesterol
— indigestion
— irritable bowel syndrome
— liver dysfunction
— mood swings
— multiple allergic response syndrome (MARS)
— multiple food allergies
— muscle or joint pain
— nausea and bloating
— premenstrual syndrome (PMS)
— prostate disorders
— sinus infections
— sluggish lymphatic system
— sore or bleeding gums
— yeast infections or vaginitis

Score 1 point for each symptom/illness checked. Add the total here _____. Now divide this number by 40 and multiply the answer by 100. Write the final number here _____.

Section E

— acne, blackheads, or whiteheads
— blotchy or ruddy skin
— dry and/or flaky skin
— dry, scaly patches of skin
— eczema
— hives
— psoriasis
— rashes

Score 1 point for each symptom/illness checked. Add the total here _____. Now divide this number by 8 and multiply the answer by 100. Write the final number here _____.

Once you've totaled your responses in each section and multiplied the total by the number specified, circle the section with the highest score: Section A B C D E.

Interpreting Your Quiz Results

The quiz results can help point you in the direction of the best detox for you based on your symptoms. Now check the section you circled against the chart below, which points to the Weekend Wonder Detox that you may wish to start using. Of course, you can select any of the detoxes that interest you. If you really want a jumpstart on losing weight, for example, you can start with the Fat Blast Weekend. Or, if you have recurring urinary tract infections, you can jump right to the Kidney Flush Weekend. If your skin condition bothers you, you can dive right into the Skin Rejuvenation Weekend. If you suffer from a lot of muscle or joint pain, try the Lymphomania Weekend. If you tend toward constipation, choose the Colon Cleanse Weekend. The Love Your Liver Weekend is always a good idea because it is the main organ that processes all those toxins we discussed in Chapter 1. If you really aren't sure where to begin even after taking the quiz, that's no problem—the Love Your Liver Weekend is a good overall cleanse to give your body a much-needed boost.

Section A—The Love Your Liver Weekend
Section B—The Lymphomania Weekend
Section C—The Kidney Flush Weekend
Section D—The Colon Cleanse Weekend
Section E—The Skin Rejuvenation Weekend

If your score on the quiz has you down, don't worry. These weekends are designed to help you transform your health, looks, and, yes, your whole life.

Each of the weekend detoxes builds on the essentials outlined in this chapter, so be sure to read the rest of this chapter before moving on to the specific detox you've chosen.

THE ESSENTIALS FOR ALL THE WEEKEND WONDER DETOXES

Some elements of the detox weekends are the same regardless of which one you choose. Below I've outlined the dietary guidelines that you should follow no matter which detox you're doing. In the following chapters you'll discover additional eating guidelines, detox superfoods that target a particular organ, specific nutrients and herbs that boost your efforts, and targeted exercises and spa treatments for the particular detox you've selected. For example, if you select the Love Your Liver Weekend, you'll follow all of the essentials below, plus those outlined in Chapter 3. If you select the Fat Blast Weekend, you'll follow the essentials below and the various instructions in Chapter 8.

Eliminate the Three Ps:
It's Not Really Food, So Your Body Won't Miss It

The consumption of processed, packaged, or prepared foods (I use that term loosely here) can derail any commitment to health, including a weekend wonder detox. Yes, there are some good, healthy products that come in boxes, bags, or cans; however, the vast majority of the foods you find in containers are loaded with chemicals and nonfood substances that are toxic, addictive, or both. Your body is not designed to consume or digest these "nonfoods," and yet they make up an alarming percentage of the standard diet. We have become accustomed to eating these substances and think nothing of it. Their addictive properties make us believe they are among our favorite foods.

Avoid the 3Ps and you'll automatically be avoiding most food additives, colors, artificial sweeteners, preservatives, or harmful fats. Your liver, kidneys, intestines, lymphatic system, and skin need to detoxify your body of all of these synthetic food additives. Many of these toxins are also stored in fat. Eating them during this weekend will simply negate your best efforts. For this weekend, and even afterward if you are so inclined, eliminate processed foods, artificial food additives, colors, and preservatives from your diet along with the 3Ps: processed, prepared, and packaged foods.

Of course, you'll need to read ingredient lists on any packaged foods you purchase. But remember that not all harmful ingredients are listed, and some are listed under alternate names (recall our discussion of MSG in Chapter 1).

Nix Sugar and Other Sweeteners

During the detox weekends you'll want to avoid all refined sugar, artificial sweeteners, and even so-called healthier sweetening options. The average person eats more than two and a half pounds of sugar each week, so reducing your consumption for three days can help your body recover from this sugary onslaught. Ideally, I encourage you to reduce your consumption significantly after that too. But start with three days. If you're moaning that you can't possibly do it, then you are seriously in need of eliminating it, as this reaction typically points to a sugar addiction.

Give your body a much-needed break from sugars and sugar substitutes by eliminating white sugar, brown sugar, demerara sugar, dehydrated cane juice, honey, maple syrup, molasses, beet sugar, coconut sugar, palm sugar, agave nectar, rice malt, fructose, corn syrup, aspartame, sucralose, saccharin, and any other concentrated sweeteners.

There is one sweetener that's fine to use: stevia drops, which are naturally hundreds of times sweeter than sugar. Unlike other concentrated sweeteners, stevia does not affect blood sugar levels. You can also use the herb in its dried and powdered form; however, this form has a slightly bitter taste that doesn't appeal to everyone. Also be aware that there are many companies corrupting stevia with harmful ingredients and other sweeteners. I find that the liquid stevia tends to be purer and usually tastes better than the powder. If you're using the drops, just two or three will taste as sweet as the equivalent number of teaspoons of sugar. If you choose the dried, powdered form, a pinch will do. Keep in mind that I'm not talking about the white, powdered stevia that is diluted with maltodextrin, dextrose, or other sweeteners that are not allowed on the Weekend Wonder Detox.

A moderate amount of fresh fruit is fine throughout the Weekend Wonder Detoxes except during the Fat Blast Weekend. Fruit is nature's cleanser, but some people are vulnerable to weight gain if they eat excess amounts.

You may notice a small amount of honey is used in some of the recipes in this book. A teaspoon at a time up to three times daily is fine. Choose local, unpasteurized honey for this purpose.

Skip the Soda

Now that we've discussed the importance of eliminating sugars and artificial sweeteners, I probably don't need to tell you that includes soda. A typical soda really shouldn't be classified as a food; it's more of a toxic waste dump in a can. Yet the average person guzzles fifty-three gallons of soda every year—that's a whopping 848 cups annually. If you did only one great thing for your health, it would be to pass on the soda. Studies show that phosphoric acid leaches calcium and other minerals from our bones and teeth, prevents mineral absorption, and contributes to osteoporosis.[1] Each can of soda contains eleven teaspoons of sugar—that's excessive by anyone's standards. So if you haven't already cut out the soda, now is the time. Do not drink any soda on the Weekend Wonder Detox. This includes diet soda, regular soda, fruit soda, or carbonated water. (If you're wondering about diet soda, remember our discussion of artificial sweeteners—diet soda is not a healthy drink!)

Ditch Dairy

During the Weekend Wonder Detox you choose it is important to eliminate dairy from your diet. Dairy is mucous forming and can clog the body's natural detoxification processes. Besides that, today's dairy products are simply not the health foods we've been taught they are, for many reasons.

Cow's milk is intended for baby cows. We're the only species, other than those we domesticate, that drinks milk after infancy. And we're definitely the only ones drinking the milk of a different species. Baby cows have four stomachs to digest milk. We have one.

Dairy products contain hormones. Not only are the naturally present hormones in cow's milk stronger than human hormones, but the animals are also routinely given steroids and other hormones to plump them up and increase milk production. These hormones can negatively affect humans' delicate hormonal balance.

Most cows are fed inappropriate food. Commercial feed for cows contains all sorts of ingredients that include genetically modified (GM) corn, GM soy, animal products, chicken manure, cottonseed, pesticides, and antibiotics. Guess what that feed becomes? Your milk.

Research shows that the countries whose citizens consume the most dairy products have the *highest* incidence of osteoporosis, contrary to what dairy bureaus try to tell us.

Research links dairy products with the formation of arthritis. In one study on rabbits, scientist Richard Panush was able to *produce* inflamed joints in the animals by switching their water to milk. In another study scientists observed more than a 50 percent reduction in the pain and swelling of arthritis when participants eliminated milk and dairy products from their diet.

Most dairy products are pasteurized to kill potentially harmful bacteria. During the pasteurization process, however, vitamins, proteins, and enzymes are destroyed. Enzymes assist with the digestion process. When they are destroyed through pasteurization, milk becomes harder to digest, therefore putting a strain on our bodies' enzyme systems.

Most milk is homogenized, which denatures the milk's proteins, making it harder to digest. Many peoples' bodies react to these proteins as though they are "foreign invaders," causing their immune systems to overreact.

Further, pesticides in cow feed find their way into milk and dairy products that we consume. As you learned in the last chapter, pesticides are harmful neurotoxins that can be damaging to our bodies.

Meat of the Matter

During the Weekend Wonder Detox avoid eating meat. I'm not suggesting that you have to be vegan for the rest of your life. Most meat contains antibiotics, hormones, and arachidonic acid, which is healthy in smaller amounts but causes inflammation when consumed in excess. Arachidonic acid is a type of Omega 6 fatty acid that the body requires. But most people eat about twenty to forty times as much Omega 6 fatty acids as they do anti-inflammatory Omega 3s, and it is the ratio here that is the issue. One of the main reasons this ratio is disproportionate is that most people are eating way too much meat. In the quantities most people eat it, Omega 6 fatty acids cause inflammation, which is linked to many chronic illnesses, including allergies, arthritis, cancer, diabetes, and heart disease.

Meat also takes a fair amount of time and energy to digest. For the detox we want to free up that energy for cleansing and healing and to restore a healthy Omega fatty acid balance. So go ahead and eat meat, preferably organic, *after* the cleanse is over if you want, but for now it is best avoided. That includes beef, bison, chicken, duck, lamb, pork, and turkey.

So you've learned about many of the foods and food additives to avoid, but it's equally important to eat healthy food during the Weekend Wonder Detox. After all, the foods you eat are broken down into their components like amino acids, fatty acids, vitamins, minerals, and sugars to create the cells, tissues, organs, and organ systems in your body. That's why it is essential to eat high-quality, nutrient-dense foods free from toxins.

A Detox Fish Tale

Many types of fish are high in the Omega 3 fatty acids known as eicosapentanoic acid (EPA) and docosahexanoic acid (DHA), both of which are beneficial to a healthy brain and nervous system as well as healthy joints. Because of their anti-inflammatory nature, they can reduce the inflammation that has been linked with many serious illnesses.

But not all fish are beneficial. Some contain high amounts of pollutants like mercury and pesticides. Although mackerel and tuna are often recommended due to their high Omega 3 content, they are also frequently high in mercury, so it's best to avoid them. You'll also want to skip seafood because many are bottom-feeders that tend to have higher levels of pollutants.

Some of the fish that regularly tests low in these harmful substances and high in Omega 3 fatty acids include wild salmon, anchovies, sardines, lake trout, and herring.

These fish are okay to eat while on the Weekend Wonder Detox.

A Grain of Truth

You'll need to avoid all refined grains like white flour and white rice during the Weekend Wonder Detox. You can still eat many whole grains, but I encourage people to stick to the gluten-free options, particularly if you're suffering from any health condition or are overweight. Gluten is a type of protein found in many grains. The industrialization and hybridization of many grain crops have resulted in grains that are higher in gluten than would naturally have appeared; many ancient grains like kamut tend to be naturally lower in gluten. Regardless, if you have a gluten sensitivity or a full-blown gluten allergy, then it doesn't matter how much gluten these grains contain. It's like poison to a person with gluten sensitivity and especially to those with gluten allergies or celiac disease.

Fortunately, there are many gluten-free grains that you can enjoy on the Weekend Wonder Detox. Here are six gluten-free grains you can add to your diet.

Brown Rice
Unlike white rice, brown rice is high in fiber and vitamin E. Vitamin E is essential for healthy skin, immune function, and many other critical functions in your body. During the processing of brown rice into white, however, these nutrients are largely lost. Brown rice contains high amounts of the minerals manganese,

magnesium, and selenium. It also contains tryptophan, which helps with sleep quality. Selenium helps ward off cancer. Brown rice can easily replace white rice in almost any recipe—soups, stews, stir-fries—and can even be used to make a dairy-free milk substitute, and it is definitely allowed on the Weekend Wonder Detox.

Buckwheat

The name is a bit misleading. Buckwheat is *not* related to wheat and is both wheat- and gluten-free. It's not even technically a grain but a seed that's a relative of rhubarb, but that's another story. It is high in fiber, manganese, magnesium, tryptophan, and copper. Research shows that the regular consumption of buckwheat reduces the incidence of high blood pressure and high cholesterol. The combination of vitamin C and the flavonoid rutin give buckwheat its ability to prevent blood clumping and to keep blood moving smoothly through blood vessels. Canadian research in the *Journal of Agriculture and Food Chemistry* found that buckwheat may be helpful in managing diabetes.

Millet

Similar in texture to couscous, millet is high in manganese, phosphorus, tryptophan, and magnesium. Phosphorus is a key component of ATP—your body's energy currency. ATP helps ensure that your body has the energy it needs for every function. Tryptophan is the amino acid that helps your body make melatonin, which in turn helps you sleep like a baby at night. Magnesium has been shown in studies to reduce the severity of headaches and asthma. And, according to new research published in the *American Journal of Gastroenterology*, foods high in insoluble fiber like millet can help reduce the incidence of gallstones.

Gluten-Free Oats

Not all oats are gluten-free, but certain gluten-free varieties are currently being marketed. If you have a severe gluten sensitivity or intolerance, gluten-free oats may not be right for you; however, they are fine for most people. They help stabilize blood sugar and lower cholesterol and are high in protein and fiber. Oats are available in many forms, including instant, steel-cut, rolled, bran, groats, flakes, and flour. The best options are the less refined ones like steel-cut, rolled, flakes, and bran. Gluten-free oat flour is an excellent substitute for wheat flour in baking recipes. It is a good source of minerals like manganese, selenium, magnesium, and the sleep aid tryptophan, and, according to many studies, oats also assist with lowering cholesterol and reducing the risk of heart disease.

Quinoa

Quinoa, a staple of the ancient Incas who revered it as sacred, is not a true grain; rather, it is the seed of an herb. Unlike most grains, quinoa is a complete protein (other grains are missing essential amino acids and are therefore not complete proteins) and is high in iron, magnesium, B-vitamins, and fiber. In studies quinoa is a proven aid for migraine sufferers and, like most whole grains, lessens the risk for heart disease. It also contains the building blocks for superoxide dismutase, an important antioxidant that helps protect the energy centers of your cells from free-radical damage. Quinoa cooks in fifteen minutes, making it the ultimate supernutritious fast food.

Wild Rice

Like millet and quinoa, wild rice is not a true grain; it's actually a type of aquatic grass seed native to the United States and Canada. It tends to be a bit pricier than other grains, but its high content of protein and nutty flavor make wild rice worth every penny. It's an excellent choice for people with celiac disease or those who have gluten or wheat sensitivities. Wild rice also has a lower caloric content than many grains, at only 83 calories per half cup of cooked rice. And it is high in fiber. Add wild rice to soups, stews, salads, and pilaf. It's important to note that wild rice is black. There are many blends of white and wild rice, which primarily consist of refined white rice—be sure to use only real wild rice, not the blends.

Salt of the Earth

Iodized salt is heavily processed and nutritionally dead. Instead, choose unrefined sea salt. Some people suggest crystal salt, but that often has excessive amounts of lead, which can be dangerous to your health. I prefer unrefined sea salt, which has a grayish color, reflecting the many minerals, not just sodium, it contains. Use it in moderation only.

Go Organic

Eat organic foods throughout the Weekend Wonder Detox. In study after study it shows up as being more nutritious, plus you'll reduce your exposure to pesticides, herbicides, fungicides, genetically modified organisms (GMOs), and much more. Ideally, keep eating organic food after the detox too. Here are fourteen reasons why I recommend eating organic food as much as possible and throughout the Weekend Wonder Detox:

Fourteen Essential Reasons to Eat Organic Food

1. Genetically modified foods were unleashed on the environment and the public by corporations like Monsanto without prior testing to determine their safety. In other words, eating genetically modified foods (which most people ingest in large amounts) is participating in a long-term, uncontrolled experiment. Choose organic to avoid participation in this experiment. As you learned in Chapter 1, more and more research is coming in about the health threat of genetically modified food. The results range from intestinal damage, allergies, liver or pancreatic problems, testicular cellular changes, tumors, and even death in the experimental animals. Eating third-party-certified organic foods or those that are guaranteed to be grown from organic seed helps protect you from the health consequences of GMOs.

2. In study after study research from independent organizations consistently shows organic food is higher in nutrients than

traditional foods. Research shows that organic produce is higher in vitamin C, antioxidants, and the minerals calcium, iron, chromium, and magnesium. (For more information, check out my book *The Life Force Diet*).

3. They're free of neurotoxins, which are damaging to brain and nerve cells. A commonly used class of pesticides called organophosphates was originally developed as a toxic nerve agent during World War I. When there was no longer a need for them in warfare, industry adapted them to kill pests on plants. Many pesticides are still considered neurotoxins.

4. Children's growing brains and bodies are far more susceptible to toxins than those of adults. Choosing organic helps feed their bodies without exposing them to pesticides and genetically modified organisms.

5. Eighteen percent of all genetically modified seeds (and, therefore, foods that grow from them) are engineered to produce their own pesticides. Research shows that these seeds continue producing pesticides inside your body once you've eaten the food grown from them! Foods that are actually pesticide factories . . . no, thanks.

6. The US Environmental Protection Agency (EPA) estimates that pesticides pollute the primary drinking source for half the American population. Organic farming is the best solution to the problem. Buying organic helps reduce pollution in our drinking water.

7. Organic food is earth supportive (when big business keeps their hands out of it). Organic food production has been around for thousands of years and is the sustainable choice for the future. Compare that to modern agricultural practices that are destroying the environment through widespread use of herbicides, pesticides, fungicides, and fertilizers and have resulted in drastic environmental damage in many parts of the world.

8. Organic food choices grown on small-scale organic farms help ensure independent family farmers can create a livelihood. Consider it the domestic version of fair trade.

9. Most organic food simply tastes better than the pesticide-grown counterparts.

10. Organic farms are safer for farm workers. Research at the Harvard School of Public Health found a 70 percent increase in Parkinson's disease among people exposed to pesticides. Choosing organic foods means that more people will be able to work on farms without incurring the higher potential health risk of Parkinson's or other illnesses.

11. Organic food supports wildlife habitats. Even with commonly used amounts of pesticides, exposure to pesticides is harming wildlife.

12. Eating organic may reduce your cancer risk. The US Environmental Protection Agency (EPA) considers 60 percent of herbicides, 90 percent of fungicides, and 30 percent of insecticides potentially cancer causing. It is reasonable to think that the rapidly increasing rates of cancer are at least partly linked to the use of these carcinogenic pesticides.

13. Choosing organic meat lessens your exposure to antibiotics, synthetic hormones, and drugs that find their way into the animals and, ultimately, into you.

14. Organic food supports greater biodiversity. Diversity is fundamental to life on this planet. Genetically modified and non-organic food is focused on high-yield monoculture and is destroying biodiversity. For example, there are hundreds, if not thousands of types of organic heirloom tomatoes that evolved over time for superior taste and nutrition, yet we see only a couple of varieties in most grocery stores. The latter varieties tend to be attractive to consumers but are nutritionally inferior to the heirloom varieties.

Water, Water, Everywhere . . . and Required by Every Cell

We constantly hear about the importance of drinking enough water. On the flip side there has been a growing trend in the media lately touting that the recommended eight cups of water daily is a myth, which is technically accurate but not the whole story. Whether you need eight cups of water daily or ten or even fourteen, most people are not getting the message that whatever their particular water needs are, they aren't meeting them.

And even dieticians, nutritionists, and medical professionals are contributing to the problem by informing people that they get enough water in their diet in the form of fruits and vegetables. That might be true for some people, but, after assessing the diets of countless people, I assure you that isn't the case for most people. Plus, have you ever noticed that when you throw vegetables in a pan and turn on the heat you'll see liquid in the pan soon afterward, and then shortly after that you'll see steam rising from them? That's because you're literally cooking the water out of the vegetables.

Researchers estimate that half of the world's population is chronically dehydrated. And in America that level is even higher, at 75 percent of the population. In my experience most people who are experiencing pain or illness are chronically dehydrated. It's that simple.

More than two-thirds of your body weight is water. Every cell and organ requires adequate water to function properly. Without adequate water your body's biochemical and electrical (yes, electrical—read on!) functions begin to break down. The list of reasons your body needs water is as plentiful as the functions in your body, so due to space limitations, here are eleven good reasons to drink more water.

1. Your blood is over 80 percent water and needs water to make healthy new blood cells.
2. Your bones are over 50 percent water and, you guessed it, need water to make healthy new bone cells.
3. Drinking more water actually helps lessen pain in your body by getting your lymphatic system moving. The lymphatic system is a network of nodes, tubes, and vessels that move waste out of your tissues. It requires water to function properly.

4. Water helps to eliminate wastes and toxins from your body through the lymphatic system, kidneys, and intestines.
5. Water lubricates your joints and helps reduce joint pain.
6. Water regulates metabolism, so, if you're overweight, chances are you may need more water.
7. Water balances body temperature.
8. Water helps to ensure adequate electrical functioning so our brain and nervous system function properly.
9. Every cell and organ requires adequate water to function properly.
10. Water alleviates dehydration—and we already established that most people are chronically dehydrated.
11. And water is critical for healthy detoxification. Without sufficient water, toxins can get backed up in your liver, cannot be flushed from your kidneys, will be absorbed into your blood through the walls of your intestines, get backed up in your lymphatic system, cannot be eliminated via the skin, and will not be broken down from fat stores in your body.

So one of the quickest and easiest ways to detoxify is to start drinking more pure water every day. In wealthy, developed nations with plentiful access to water, we really have no excuses for not drinking enough. If possible, purchase an inexpensive water filtration system. For long-term use I recommend getting a counter top model but, if that's not in your budget, even a water filtration pitcher will help. But they are not all created equally.

During your Weekend Wonder Detox drink at least one-half quart or one-half liter (almost the same amount) for every fifty pounds of weight you're carrying, up to about three quarts or liters. I know this seems like a lot (because it is!), and you may feel like you're spending your weekend in the bathroom, but your body needs water to flush toxins out. We don't want all the toxins we're digging up to be absorbed back into your bloodstream, creating a vicious cycle of sloughing off toxins only to have them be reabsorbed into the blood.

Super Salads for Super Health

Regardless which detox you choose, you'll want to eat plenty of salads throughout the weekend. I'm not talking about potato salad, macaroni salad, or Jell-O salad here—salads full of leafy greens and other raw veggies and sprouts, because they are full of plant nutrients and enzymes that aid detoxification. Eat at least one large salad daily while doing the detox, but preferably more. On page 254 in the Recipe section I've included a chart to help you create delicious gourmet, health-promoting salads in minutes. If the thought of salads causes you to recoil in disgust, the chart will help you transform your thinking about salads.

The Veggies Have It

Focus on vegetables at every meal. Whether you choose veggie juices, add a handful of leafy greens to your smoothie, or sauté a plate of vegetables for your dinner, vegetables should always be the focal point of meals during the Weekend Wonder Detox.

If you don't like vegetables, you simply haven't found a way to prepare them to change this view. My husband wasn't a big fan of vegetables when we met, but now he regularly chooses veggie-rich meals as his favorites. Even the most hated of vegetables can taste great if you top them with a delicious marinade or sauté them with some garlic and a pinch of sea salt. I've never been a big fan of green beans, but sauté them with garlic, a touch of olive oil, and a pinch of sea salt, and they transform into one of my favorites. You'll need to be creative to find ways to love vegetables. But if you're not feeling so creative, just flip to the Recipe section of this book to find delicious and nutritious vegetable recipes that satisfy your palate while you satisfy your cells.

There are so many vegetables to choose from, so be sure to mix it up a bit. One of the best things you can do for your health is to eat more vegetables and a wide variety of them. Each one contains a nutrient profile that is unlike any other, so eating a variety helps to ensure you get all the nutrients your body needs and lots of phy-tonutrients (plant nutrients) that provide optimum health.

Sprout Out Loud

If you haven't tried sprouts—and there are a lot more kinds than just alfalfa!—then I urge you to do so on the Weekend Wonder Detox. Impressive things happen to a seed when it begins to sprout, and all of these things mean better nutrition for your body. Here are some of the nutritional transformations that occur:

1. **Vitamin content in seeds multiplies.** This is especially true of vitamins A, C, E, and the B-complex vitamins. The vitamin content of some beans, seeds, or grains can increase by up to twenty times its original value within only a few days of sprouting. Research shows that the sprouting process increases vitamins B1 up to 285 percent, B2 up to 515 percent, and niacin up to 256 percent.[2]

2. **The quality of protein in the bean, grain, or seed improves.** The proteins change form during soaking and sprouting, thereby improving its nutritional value. For example, the amino acid lysine, which is critical to prevent cold sores and to maintain healthy immunity, increases during this process.[3]

3. **Essential fatty acid content increases during the sprouting process.** These are the healthy fats our bodies need to ensure healthy skin, hair, brain, immune system, and more.[4]

4. **Fiber content increases substantially.** In a study fiber content almost doubled during the sprouting of one type of seed.[5] We need fiber to push toxins out of our intestines, so getting more fiber is valuable on the Weekend Wonder Detox.

5. **Enzyme content multiplies.** Enzymes are special types of proteins that aid digestion and metabolism, among other things. When sprouts are eaten in their natural, raw state your body benefits from the enzyme increase through improved digestion and energy.

If you haven't eaten many sprouts, here are some easy ways to incorporate them into your diet: add clover or alfalfa sprouts to a wrap, use mung bean sprouts as the base for an Asian-inspired salad, add a handful of any type of sprout to your favorite salad recipe, throw a handful of mung bean sprouts on your favorite noodle dish or stir-fry after it has finished cooking, or spice up a salad or wrap with mustard or radish sprouts. Be creative. Sprouts are delicious. If you don't like one type, try another. And try them in different ways.

Some people have expressed concern that they read about sprouts causing food poisoning. Any food can cause food poisoning, and sprouts are no more vulnerable than any other type of food; however, people often skip washing sprouts, making the chance of food poisoning greater. Always wash your sprouts, just as you should with all produce.

Eat as many sprouts as you'd like. They are the most overlooked and inexpensive superfoods.

Not Forbidden Fruit

Fruit is Nature's cleansing food; you'll enjoy a wide variety of it on the Weekend Wonder Detox. However, there may be specific limitations to type and amount listed in the individual detox recommendations in the next six chapters. If you're watching your weight or trying to lose weight, you'll want to be mindful of how much extremely sweet fruit you eat, including bananas, pineapples, and grapes, to name a few. The natural sugars in fruit are great to boost energy, but they can be turned into fat if eaten in excess.

Bean Around the World

You can enjoy many legumes and beans on the Weekend Wonder Detox. I encourage you to eat them daily. Beans are high in fiber and a good source of protein. They help clear the bowels, and they bind to toxins to escort them out of your body. Feel free to enjoy beans of all kinds—chickpeas, edamame (green soy beans), kidney beans, lentils, lima beans, navy beans, pinto beans, romano beans, soy beans, and more. If you're buying canned beans, choose ones free of EDTA and packaged in BPA-free cans. Read labels to be sure.

Nuts About Nuts and Seeds

Choose raw, unsalted nuts and seeds, preferably found in the refrigerator section of your local health food store. Due to their high oil content, nuts and seeds can be vulnerable to heat, light, and lengthy storage so it's important to get good, fresh nuts. Feel free to enjoy many types of nuts, including almonds, Brazil nuts, cashews, hazelnuts, pecans, pistachios, and walnuts. You can also enjoy many types of seeds, including chia seeds, flax seeds, hemp seeds, pumpkin seeds, sesame seeds, and sunflower seeds. Chia seeds can be added to smoothies for an instant boost of fiber, protein, and hormone-balancing compounds. Flax seeds and hemp seeds should never be heated but can be sprinkled on top of food after it has been cooked or added to smoothies. It's best to freshly grind flax seeds to obtain their oils, as the whole seeds tend to go through the digestive tract intact.

Although the nutritional composition of nuts and seeds varies greatly, all nuts and seeds tend to be high in protein, which is needed for healthy skin, hair, nails, and tissue growth. Some nuts and seeds, such as chia, flax, walnuts, and pumpkin seeds, tend to be high in Omega 3 fatty acids, making them valuable for strong immunity, wrinkle- and blemish-free skin, and many other functions in your body.

As stated above, be sure to choose fresh, raw nuts found in the refrigerator section of your local health food or grocery store. The essential fatty acids found in nuts and seeds go rancid easily, and eating rancid nuts and seeds exposes your body to further toxins that wreak havoc on cells. Eating fresh, raw nuts and seeds provides your body with essential building blocks for health and life. Plus, they taste better.

Got Milk Substitutes?

Because there are no dairy products included on the Weekend Wonder Detox, you may be wondering what you can use in place of milk. There are many great delicious, nutritious, and easy-to-use alternatives: almond, coconut, hemp, rice, or organic soy milk (the latter in moderation only, and only if it is certified organic). Read labels, though, as many manufacturers add ingredients that are less than healthful; some manufacturers add preservatives and gums to thicken them. Choose unsweetened varieties. If you prefer them sweeter tasting, add a couple of drops of liquid stevia when using.

Give Your Body an Oil Change

You can use coconut oil or extra virgin olive oil for cooking or in place of butter or margarine. With extra virgin olive oil be sure not to heat it too high, as it begins to smoke around 325 degrees. Coconut oil can handle slightly higher heat, but you should still avoid overheating it. When an oil is heated above its smoke point, it loses its beneficial properties and instead can cause inflammation. If the oil smokes, throw it out. Cook on low to medium heat to avoid this problem. It may take some time to get used to cooking on low to medium temperatures, as the food takes a bit longer, but your health is worth it.

You can add flax seed oil, hempseed oil, sesame oil, or sunflower oil to your food. The former two should not be heated to keep the natural oils intact. Regardless which type of oil you choose, be sure it is cold-pressed, because most grocery store oils have been excessively heated and do not have a place on the Weekend Wonder Detox. Try to avoid them afterward as well.

Spice Up Your Life

Almost all spices can be used on the Weekend Wonder Detox. Actually I encourage you to use spices to give your food flavor.

Most spices are packed with phytonutrients that ward off bacteria, viruses, fungi, and cancer, and they fend off many health issues. Feel free to use basil, cardamom, celery seed (use it like salt), chili peppers, cilantro, cinnamon, cloves, cumin, ginger, oregano, parsley, rosemary, sage, thyme, turmeric, and many others. Remember: fresh is always best. But if you can't find fresh spices, dried ones are fine. The only ones you should avoid are ones that have been irradiated, which includes most dried spices sold in grocery stores. Choose organic if possible, as they tend not to be irradiated.

Eat Small and Often

I know many people who eat extremely healthy but skip meals, eat on the run, or avoid eating for hours at a time. Skipping meals or not eating often enough is as unhealthy as eating junk food. Your body needs food every two to three hours to help maintain stable blood sugar levels. Stable blood sugar ensures that your brain and every part of your body have the energy they need to function properly. Skipping meals or eating infrequently causes weight gain, mood swings, and energy crashes, and it can aggravate pain conditions and other health issues.

While following the Weekend Wonder Detox be sure to eat or snack every two to three hours. (I'll give you lots of snack suggestions each weekend and in the Recipe section.) You shouldn't eat so much that you feel heavy and bloated. Smaller is better when it comes to portions on a detox, but don't use detoxification as an excuse to undereat either.

Multi-ply Your Detox Success

Taking a high-quality multivitamin and mineral supplement throughout your detox weekends will help you avoid any deficiencies. The various processes of detoxification in the liver, kidneys, lymphatic system, skin, colon, and even in fat stores depend on many nutrients to detoxify properly. Even a single nutrient deficiency can be harmful and cause a malfunction in detoxification, so it's important to give your body a boost with a good, quality multivitamin. It should contain only naturally sourced nutrients and be free of colors, sweeteners, artificial sweeteners, fillers, preservatives, gluten, and allergens like corn, soy, and wheat. Always consult with a naturally minded physician before starting any new supplements.

Herbs: Nature's Potent Remedies

Herbs are included for each of the Weekend Wonder Detoxes. They are specific to the selected detox. The herbs recommended for the liver detox will vary greatly from the herbs recommended for the lymphatic system herbs, and so on. So stick with the herbs recommended for the specific cleanse you select.

Whenever I mention herbs throughout the *Weekend Wonder Detox* you'll notice that I've included the scientific names. That's to ensure you are obtaining the correct herb when you visit your local herbal dispensary, natural food store, or health professional. Don't worry—you don't need to purchase all of the herbs mentioned in each detox; one to three is sufficient. I've included extra ones, should you have difficulty finding any of the herbs in stores. You'll also find some herbal tea blends in the Recipe section of this book. If you make these herbal teas and drink them three times daily, you won't need to take the additional recommended capsules or herbal products in each detox. Most of the herbs can be found at your local health food store.

Be sure to choose organic or "wild-crafted" herbs because you don't want ones that have been sprayed with pesticides or other toxins, which would be counterproductive on the detox. All of the herbs I recommend are proven through scientific studies and/or a lengthy and safe history of use when used as directed.

If you are picking your own wild herbal medicines, be sure that you have sufficient knowledge to identify them properly. Also, be sure to avoid herbs near roadsides or polluted or industrial areas.

Of course, you don't need to pick them yourself, as most health food stores have them in dried, capsule, or tincture (alcohol-extract) form.

Although alcohol extracts are great, I advise you to choose one of the other forms of the herbs while doing the Love Your Liver Weekend or if you have impaired liver function, as the alcohol can be difficult for the liver if it is in a severely weakened state. The exception is milk thistle because its active ingredients are not extracted well in water or tea. Of course, steer clear of alcohol extracts if you have ever been an alcoholic or if you are diabetic.

Consult an herbalist or natural medicine specialist before taking herbs with any medications or if you suffer from a serious health condition. Avoid using herbs while pregnant or lactating, and avoid long-term use of any herb without first consulting a qualified professional.

Exercises for Detoxification

There are specific exercises recommended for each weekend detox. Some are inspired by Western systems of exercise, like cardiovascular exercise, weight training, and rebounding. The latter is a form of a gentle minitrampoline-type exercise that has been found to be particularly effective to get the lymphatic system moving but can also be used in other weekend detoxes if you would like.

Other exercises are drawn from Eastern forms of exercise like yoga and qigong. Most people are familiar with yoga as a form of stretching, strengthening, and structurally aligning exercise. Qigong (pronounced chee-gung) is less known but is a form of gentle movement that improves strength, breathing, balance, and structural alignment. Additionally, it also works to rebalance the body's energy systems. Research has shown what the Chinese have known for thousands of years, that there are energy lines in the body that connect to organs and glands and that surface at points on the skin, known as acupoints. Sometimes these points can become blocked from toxins, stress, injury, or many other reasons.

Qigong works to help disperse any blockages in the energy systems, known as meridians.

Spa Therapies for Super Cleansing

That takes me to some of the many natural healing therapies throughout Weekend Wonder Detox, including acupressure, massage, aromatherapy, meditation, and hydrotherapy (healing with water). Acupressure is based on the same knowledge of energy systems in the body as qigong—they both work to disperse energy blockages. Qigong works through stretching exercises, whereas acupressure works by using finger pressure on the acupoints to eliminate any blockages in the energy meridians. All of the spa treatments have been selected for their ability to balance your body and create an environment in which your body can heal itself.

Exercises and Spa Treatments for Each Detox
Here are some of the exercises and spa therapies you'll explore for each of the Weekend Wonder Detoxes:

Love Your Liver Weekend—You'll discover the qigong exercise called the Crane Pose, which helps to improve liver function and overall balance. You'll also experience acupressure and an aromatherapy compress that targets the liver for detoxification and healing.

The Lymphomania Weekend—For this weekend you'll explore rebounding on a minitrampoline, which helps get stagnant lymph fluid moving. Don't worry if you're not familiar with the lymphatic system yet—we'll be discussing it in detail in Chapter 4. You'll also learn a lymph-boosting massage technique and dry skin brushing, both of which assist in moving toxins out of the lymph system.

The Kidney Flush Weekend—The exercise for this detox is called the Leg Sweep and Swing, which is based on a form of yoga. It helps flush toxins, eliminate infections, and improve overall kidney health. You'll also partake of the Healthy Kidney Meditation, a form of relaxation and visualization to help restore the kidneys and urinary tract. Using gentle acupressure, you'll help to disperse any blockages that could be interfering with your kidney and urinary tract health.

The Colon Cleanse Weekend—For this weekend you'll perform Colon Cleanse Cardio and an exercise called Knees-to-Chest, which is based in yoga and helps to get the bowels moving. You'll also get in tune with your body by experiencing Acupressure Abdominal Massage, which activates key points in the abdomen that aid healthy bowel function.

The Skin Rejuvenation Weekend—During this weekend you'll experience Cardio to Heal the Skin as the exercise while enjoying many wonderful skin-soothing therapies like the Aromatherapy Skin Softener Bath or the At-Home Thalassotherapy Bath, Salt Body Scrub, and Skin Clarity Facial.

The Fat Blast Weekend—To supercharge your fat-burning systems you'll perform Metabolism-Boosting Cardio and Strength Training to Target Fatty Areas. You'll also enjoy the Aromatherapy Abdominal Massage as a way to improve circulation in the belly while targeting belly fat.

Worksheets and Grocery Lists

I've included some helpful worksheets at the end of each detox to make preparing for and doing the detox as simple as possible. You'll find a grocery list and a journal to help you get started and to observe any changes that occur while detoxing.

As you will probably notice throughout each detox, there are lots of customization options. I've done that intentionally to ensure you have a personalized plan that fits your health needs, budget, and schedule. I want you to feel like you've had the same personalized approach that my clients have.

FREQUENTLY ASKED QUESTIONS (FAQS) ABOUT DETOXIFICATION

Why should I detoxify?

Our bodies are exposed to more toxins now than ever before in history. At the same time our diet is more nutritionally depleted than ever before. Nutrients in food make up the building blocks of our cells, tissues, organs, and organ systems, so it is critical that we get sufficient nutrients to ensure the smooth functioning of our detoxification systems—that is hard to do on a deficient diet. Setting aside time to detoxify brings your attention back to your diet so you can make improvements. It also helps draw your attention to potential weak spots in your body so you can focus your body's natural healing ability to strengthen itself. If you're still not sure why you would want to detoxify, you may wish to reread Chapter 1 for a reminder.

I've heard that detoxification doesn't work. Is that true?

Your existence proves that detoxification works. Your liver, kidneys, skin, lymphatic system, lungs, and intestines slough off toxins every second of every day. If they didn't detoxify your body, you wouldn't be alive right now to read these questions! As for whether your body is helped through foods, natural remedies, and lifestyle changes—all of these things support your body's natural detoxification systems. Our bodies have mechanisms in place to eliminate toxins, but they still require a healthy diet and a supportive lifestyle to function properly. The foods, herbs, nutrients, exercises, and treatments in the Weekend Wonder Detox are either backed by volumes of research or have been used with success for many years, or both.

Is it safe for everyone to detoxify?

It is safe for most people to go on a detoxification regime, but not everyone should. Pregnant and nursing women should not follow a detox because their babies may be subjected to higher amounts of toxins. Diabetics and anyone with a serious health condition should not detoxify unless they have received approval from their physician and are followed by a qualified health practitioner. Even in that case, diabetics should be eating real food on a regular basis when detoxifying to avoid the potential blood sugar spikes that can occur on juice or water fasts. Of course, the Weekend Wonder Detox is not about juice or water fasts at all; it includes lots of healthy and real food, so it is safe for almost everyone. If you are taking a medication that you require to sustain your life, you should avoid detoxifying, as it can cause the medication to be removed too quickly from your body. Check with your doctor to ensure it is safe for you to detoxify. Remember that some drugs interfere with herbs and nutritional supplements, so it is important to confirm with your pharmacist or doctor to be sure there won't be any interactions.

What's the difference between detoxification and dieting? What's the difference between detoxification and cleansing?

Diets are created to lose weight. Although the term "diet" can also mean a lifestyle, many of the fad diets you hear about, promising that you'll lose an extraordinary amount of weight in a very short period of time, are not even healthy and do not contain sufficient nutrients to support a person's nutritional needs. Detoxes are designed for occasional use to give your body a boost so it can throw off stored toxins and eliminate them from your body. Detox diets usually contain food, not just water and other liquids, and tend to focus on weight loss. The Fat Blast Weekend contained in the Weekend Wonder Detox would be considered a detox diet. The Weekend Wonder Detox is a detoxification or cleansing program. Cleanses and detoxes are different words that mean the same thing.

I am taking medication my doctor prescribed. Should I continue taking it while detoxifying?

If you are on prescription medication, you should definitely continue taking it. Some medications are needed to sustain life, and even those that don't may be needed in sufficient doses to keep a health condition under control. You should never abruptly stop taking any prescription drug. If you're taking any, make sure your doctor or pharmacist says it's fine for you to detoxify. And don't forget to check with your doctor or pharmacist to ensure there won't be any interactions between the drugs you're taking and any herbs or nutritional supplements you'll be using throughout the Weekend Wonder Detox.

Are all detox programs created equally?

No. There are great programs and there are terrible ones. Even some of the great ones are terrible for some people. Most programs indicate that they target the whole body, but they mostly target either the liver or the intestines—that's not the whole body. Some detox programs are liquid only. The Weekend Wonder Detox was designed to be health supportive and to target the specific organs most in need of detoxification. No two people are the same, so one detox doesn't work for everyone. The Weekend Wonder Detox gives you the ability to assess your needs and to select the specific program that will be best for you.

Will I feel side effects while doing the detox?

Some people will, and some people will just feel great. It depends on many factors, including how toxic your body is and how healthy you've been. Some people get some symptoms on the first or second day but feel great by day two or three, depending on the person. Other people feel lighter and have more energy from the moment they start. It's difficult to predict how your body will respond. If you're accustomed to eating a lot of sugar, dairy, or caffeine, for example, you may feel withdrawal. But the side effects are usually minor. They could include headaches, nausea, fatigue, bloating, or loose bowels.

What should I do if I start to have negative symptoms?

If you experience any of the symptoms mentioned above or any other negative symptoms like general achiness, flatulence, or any others, you should drink lots of water to help your body flush out the toxins causing the problems. If you're experiencing headaches, it may not be a detoxification side effect but a caffeine-withdrawal symptom, especially if you are accustomed to drinking coffee or tea. If that's the case, have a cup of green tea or an iced green tea lemonade (see the recipe at the back of the book). The small amount of caffeine in green tea will likely give your body enough to eliminate the headache, but it is much less than the amount of caffeine found in coffee or black tea. If you have serious symptoms, you should always go to a doctor; however, I have never had a single person report serious side effects in all the years I have been working with people to help them detoxify.

Can I keep going after the three days allotted for the Weekend Wonder Detox?

Yes, of course, you can continue. If you continue to take herbal remedies after the detox weekend is over (and I encourage you to do so), you should take one week off after three weeks of using them so your body doesn't become too accustomed to taking them. And if you plan to take them for more than a couple of months, it's a good idea to consult with a qualified herbalist. Other than that you can continue as long as you wish. Be sure to eat a well-rounded diet if you continue on the Weekend Wonder Detox. And never use this detox or any other detox program as a means to support an eating disorder or addiction.

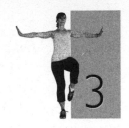

THE LOVE YOUR LIVER WEEKEND

BENEFITS OF DETOXIFYING YOUR LIVER	
• Greater energy • Clarity of thinking • Luminous skin • Flatter tummy	• Improved metabolism • Weight loss • Improved digestion

When was the last time you thought about your liver and the amazing job it's doing to filter toxins, hormones, cholesterol, and more out of your blood? Your liver is one of the most powerful organs in your body, but chances are you haven't given it a second thought. Few people consider the superorgan that sits just below their lower right ribs, working 24/7. Yet great health starts with the liver. If there was only one thing you did for your health, boosting your liver by doing the Love Your Liver Weekend would be a fantastic choice.

CLAUDIA'S BLOATING DISAPPEARS

Claudia L., a soft-spoken forty-two-year-old woman, came to my office suffering from abdominal bloating, headaches, "brain fog," fatigue, and excess weight that she found difficult to lose. Immediately I suspected that her liver was congested and needed a boost. I outlined the diet, exercises, and therapies she needed to experience a Love Your Liver Weekend detox. Eager to get started, she ran straight to the grocery store to buy the Top Ten Liver Boosting Foods and the herbs for the Liver-Enhancing Herbal Tea I recommended.

Having followed the Love Your Liver Weekend detox to the letter, she phoned me to share her experiences. Because the detox was only for three days, Claudia knew she'd have no problem sticking with the diet and exercise components. She explained that she felt a little tired and had a headache the first day, but by the end of the three days she had seen a difference in her abdomen—it was noticeably flatter. Her energy increased dramatically—something she thought was impossible, considering she had felt fatigued for years.

Claudia couldn't believe that she had a flatter stomach, felt more energetic, and had already lost four pounds after only three days but exclaimed, "If I can feel improved in only a weekend, I'm going to make Love Your Liver Weekends a monthly occurrence." She also enjoyed the Liver-Enhancing Herbal Tea and Liver Cleansing Juice so much that she wanted to keep drinking them every day. I instructed her to take a week off the Liver-Enhancing Herbal tea every three weeks so the herbs would have maximum effectiveness but to keep up her great work. I don't think she needed any reassurances, though, as her health improvements were the best motivator.

Once you experience the Love Your Liver Weekend detox I'm sure you'll understand why Claudia was so excited about her health improvements. Experiencing the detox is the best way to understand why the liver is so important.

WHY SHOULD I DETOXIFY MY LIVER?

Next to the heart and brain, the liver is arguably the most important organ in your body. With over five hundred functions to perform, it's also one of the most overworked. Some of these functions include storing vitamins, minerals, and sugars for use as fuel; controlling the production and excretion of cholesterol; and creating thousands of enzymes that control almost every function in your body. It helps your body break down fat, proteins, and carbohydrates and processes haemoglobin in the blood to allow it to use iron. It performs more biochemical tasks than any other organ in your body.

Our modern lifestyle monumentally adds to the liver's workload. The liver must filter any foreign substance that enters your body, including alcohol, tobacco, environmental pollutants, food additives, common cosmetic ingredients, household products, pharmaceutical and over-the-counter (OTC) drugs, caffeine, and food additives. It must also process internally created substances like byproducts of metabolizing food, stress or sex hormones, and much more.

The average person consumes fourteen pounds of food preservatives, additives, waxes, colors, flavors, and pesticide residues each year![1] Guess whose job it is to filter out all those potentially harmful substances? That's right: the liver. Your liver filters all these chemicals and many more. Whenever you take an antibiotic for a bacterial infection you're experiencing, the liver must filter it. When you pop an acetaminophen tablet to reduce a headache, the liver filters it. Actually, acetaminophen is also one of the worst liver-harming culprits. It can seriously damage your liver's ability to perform its many functions, leaving you feeling less than great. But I'm getting ahead of myself.

The liver simply cannot handle the onslaught of toxic chemicals and harmful substances we throw at it. Yes, most of us do so unknowingly, but the liver-damaging effects are the same. In the Love Your Liver Weekend detox you'll discover many liver-harming substances to start removing from your life, the top liver-healing foods to add to your diet, safe herbal medicines that have a proven history of healing the liver, and many natural therapies that I'll soon share.

If you did only one detox in the Weekend Wonder Detox, I would encourage you to choose the Love Your Liver Weekend. That's because cleansing and strengthening your liver can have some profound effects on your health and well-being.

SIGNS OF A STRESSED-OUT LIVER

You don't have to be diagnosed with a serious liver condition like hepatitis, jaundice, or fatty liver to have the signs of a stressed-out liver. Everyone's body is different, so you may have only one symptom or you may have a handful or more. Check out the text box that follows to see some of the signs and symptoms of a stressed-out liver.

Most people are surprised that an overworked liver can be linked to so many undesirable health symptoms and conditions. But the flip side of this is that when you strengthen the liver you can also see improvements in many health conditions.

That's why I say that if there were only one organ that could transform your health, it's your liver. Tuning up this overworked organ is critical to great health. As the liver's health improves, potentially over five hundred functions the liver performs also improve.

The liver even plays a role in serious health conditions like the pain disorder fibromyalgia and the serious immune system condition chronic fatigue syndrome (CFS), which is also known as myalgic encephalomyelitis (ME). A study conducted by Dr. Scott Rigden of over two hundred patients suffering from chronic fatigue syndrome (CFS) and/or fibromyalgia found that 80 percent of sufferers of these serious disorders had significant liver impairment. He also found that as patient's liver function tests improved, so did their symptoms, suggesting a correlation between liver stress and CFS and fibromyalgia.[2] So even if there are many other causal factors involved in serious health conditions, by improving the

SIGNS YOU WOULD BENEFIT FROM A LIVER DETOX

Here are some of the symptoms and conditions that are linked to reduced liver function or an overwhelmed liver:

abdominal bloating

alcohol intolerance

allergies

arthritis

asthma

bowel infections

"brain fog"

chronic fatigue syndrome (CFS)

colitis

Crohn's disease

depression

difficulty losing weight

environmental illness or multiple chemical sensitivities

fatigue

fatty liver

fevers

fibromyalgia

fluid retention

gallbladder disease

gallstones or gravel

gastritis

headaches and migraines

hepatitis

high blood pressure

high cholesterol levels

hives

hypoglycemia (unstable blood sugar levels)

hormone imbalances

immune system disorders

indigestion

irritable bowel syndrome

mood swings

overweight or obesity

poor appetite

poor digestion

recurring nausea and/or vomiting with no known cause

skin diseases

slow metabolism

health of the liver, you will likely see improvements in seemingly unrelated health issues as well.

If you are severely ill or do not have at least one bowel movement daily, you should consider easing into the Love Your Liver Weekend detox or start with the Colon Cleanse Weekend. It's fine to take days, weeks, or even a month or two to ease into this way of eating if that's best for you. If you are having infrequent

DO YOU HAVE A FATTY LIVER?

A high-sugar and high-fat diet also put your liver at risk of becoming fatty. You may have heard of a fatty liver.

Fatty liver is also known as non-alcoholic steatorrhoeic hepatosis (NASH) or non-alcoholic fatty liver disease (NAFLD). It contains an excessive amount of fat, causing healthy liver tissue to be replaced with areas of unhealthy fats. When this happens, the liver becomes slightly enlarged and heavier. Fatty liver is a common problem, particularly in people who are overweight and over thirty.

So how do you know whether you have a fatty liver? Here are some signs you might have a fatty liver:

- You are overweight, particularly in the abdomen
- You find losing weight to be very difficult
- You may have Type 2 diabetes
- You may feel exhausted
- You may have immune system problems
- You may have elevated triglycerides or cholesterol in your blood
- You may have been diagnosed with Syndrome X or metabolic syndrome (by a physician)

It is possible to have a fatty liver without having any symptoms. Conversely, having the symptoms above doesn't necessarily ensure that you have a fatty liver. When in doubt, consult your physician. He or she can conduct tests to determine whether you have a fatty liver. If you suspect that you have a fatty liver, diet and lifestyle changes like those mentioned throughout this chapter can help.

bowel movements (less than one daily), I highly advise you to start with the Colon Cleanse Weekend before diving into the Love Your Liver Weekend. This will ensure that the intestines can adequately remove any toxins the liver sloughs off.

Your liver is so powerful that, even if it is 80 percent impaired, it will keep working. It won't be working optimally, however, and you won't feel your best at only 20 percent liver function.

Detoxifying your liver can improve its functioning. Perhaps the best thing about the liver is its incredible ability to regenerate itself if given the critical nutrients, a healthy liver rebuilding diet, liver-strengthening herbs, and natural liver-healing therapies.

THE DIET

It is essential that you follow the dietary suggestions as closely as possible for maximum benefits. The diet comprises the Ten Love Your Liver Weekend Essentials and the Top Twelve Liver-Boosting Foods.

Ten Love Your Liver Weekend Essentials

1. **Start every morning with a large glass of water with the fresh juice of one lemon.** Sorry, but Realemon or other bottled lemon juice won't do—it must be the real deal. If you can't bear the taste of the lemon water, add a few drops of pure stevia to sweeten it—it will taste like lemonade.

2. **Avoid processed, packaged, and prepared foods.** As you know, these foods are forbidden on the Weekend Wonder Detox, but I want to reiterate its importance here in the context of liver health. Because your liver needs to process any food additives, colors, artificial sweeteners, preservatives, or harmful fats, eating them during this weekend will simply negate your best efforts. Eliminating processed foods, artificial food additives, colors, and preservatives from your diet gives your liver a well-deserved break.

3. **Avoid eating large meals.** Instead, eat small meals made up of plenty of easy-to-digest foods. Your liver works tremendously hard to aid digestion. Eating smaller meals frees up energy from digestion for the liver to detoxify your body.

4. **Eat steamed vegetables and bitter greens.** The bitter greens help to cleanse the liver. The phytochemicals ("plant chemicals") in greens cause the gall bladder to release a substance called bile. Bile emulsifies fats and many toxins so the intestines are able to

eliminate them. If you are eating bitter greens like spinach, collard, chard, or dandelion, you may notice that your stool has a greenish tinge the next few days. This is nothing to worry about and is just a sign that your liver is cleansing.

5. **Eat raw salads full of greens**. Salad greens are full of chlorophyll and enzymes that assist the liver with its detoxification duties. Chlorophyll is the substance that gives leaves and vegetables their green color. The chlorophyll molecule is similar in structure to red blood cells (haemoglobin), helping the body to make healthy and clean blood. Because your liver is the main organ that filters the blood, chlorophyll helps in this regard. The enzymes found in salad greens and other raw fruits and vegetables aid digestion, allowing the liver to focus more on detoxification and less on digestion.

6. **Eat two to three raw fruits during the day, preferably on an empty stomach**. Raw fruit also contains enzymes, which are special types of proteins that aid the digestion of the foods in which they are found. Cooking kills enzymes, so eating fruit raw (and chewing it well to release the enzymes stored in the fruit) helps clean out the bowels and improve digestion. If you're trying to lose weight, skip the high-sugar fruits like pineapple and bananas.

7. **Eat whole, raw, unsalted nuts and seeds**. Nuts and seeds are excellent sources of protein. The liver needs adequate protein to function properly. Without sufficient protein, various processes that comprise liver detoxification can break down or become impaired. Some of your best options include walnuts, almonds, Brazil nuts, pumpkin seeds, sunflower seeds, or sesame seeds. The key is choosing raw and unsalted nuts and seeds. Ideally, they are found in the refrigerator section of your health food store.

8. **Avoid eating heavy, fatty foods.** They just create more work for the liver. Avoid margarine, shortening, commercial oils, or any foods made with them. The allowable fats include cold-pressed oils, raw nuts and seeds, and avocado.

9. **Avoid eating for at least three hours before bedtime.** The liver needs adequate time during the night to perform its many functions, unimpeded by other bodily processes like digestion.

10. **Drink at least one-half quart or one-half liter (almost the same amount) for every fifty pounds of weight you're carrying, up to about three quarts or liters.** Although this may be more water than you're accustomed to, it is needed to flush toxins from your body. Without adequate water, toxins can absorb back into the bloodstream. Try not to drink right before or after meals. Vegetable and fruit juices you consume count toward your total water intake. Emphasize vegetable juices over fruit juices because the latter can be high in sugars.

Dr. Michelle's Top Twelve Liver-Boosting Foods

The liver requires high amounts of vitamins and minerals to perform its many functions. As you've already learned, your diet should be high in fruits and vegetables as well as fiber-rich foods. Here is a list of my top liver-boosting foods. Try to eat at least five of these foods every day as part of the Love Your Liver Weekend. Feel free to eat more than that. Of course, you can continue eating them after your detox is over, as they are delicious and health-promoting additions to your daily diet as well. Don't worry if you've never tried these foods before—I've included many recipes in Chapter 10 to help you incorporate them into your diet.

Avocado—Research shows that avocado supercharges other foods eaten alongside it. In other words, it boosts the nutrient absorption of other foods, particularly of a group of nutrients called carotenoids. You may have heard of beta carotene (forms vitamin A in your body) and lycopene. The absorption of both of these nutrients is increased with avocado consumption.[3] Avocados contain a type of fat that is found in seafood, but not much is found in most foods found on the land. Although they have a reputation for being "high fat," the fats they contain are beneficial and even reduce inflammation in the body. This translates to many liver health-boosting properties. If you've never eaten avocado, it tastes like butter. Use it in place of butter on bread, wraps, or sandwiches, on top of a salad, or to make a delicious guacamole or veggie dip. Simply cut lengthwise around the avocado, twist slightly to release the flesh from the pit, then, using a chopping action, hit the blade of a knife against the pit, twist, and the pit will pop right out.

Beets—These purple vegetables are powerful liver-cleansing and rebuilding foods. They contain compounds that increase the liver's ability to remove damaged cells before they can become cancerous. They contain a substance called betaine, which improves digestion, allowing the liver to redirect its energy away from digestion to focus on detoxification. Beets also help purify the blood—one of the liver's many jobs—making this hardworking organ's job easier. Enjoy beets raw (grated), steamed, boiled, and in soups and stews.

Dandelion greens—Not just a weed, dandelion greens are delicious food and powerful medicine. They contain blood-building chlorophyll, which gives them their green color. They also contain bitter compounds that help cleanse the liver. Choose young dandelion greens, as they are more palatable; the older ones become extremely bitter. You can steam, sauté, or juice the greens. Roast and grind the root for a delicious coffeelike caffeine-free beverage. I love dandelion greens chopped and sautéed with some minced garlic and olive oil, then topped with some fresh lemon juice and a dash of unrefined sea salt.

Eggs—High in a substance called lecithin, eggs help the liver metabolize fats and reduce cholesterol. They also contain phosphatidylcholine and essential fatty acids that help keep liver cells healthy and prevent fatty deposits from building up, which, as you learned earlier, can cause a fatty liver. Choose organic eggs to avoid hormones and antibiotics found in most eggs that negate their liver-boosting benefits. Enjoy scrambled, soft boiled, or in many recipes found at the back of the book.

Flax seeds and flax seed oil—Flax binds to hormone receptor sites, preventing excess hormones (including synthetic xenoestrogens from plastics and other chemicals) from floating around your bloodstream. One of the liver's five hundred jobs is to filter excess hormones. By eating flax seeds and flax oil you are helping it function more efficiently. Flax seeds can be sprinkled on cereal, toast, salads, or blended into smoothies. Flax seed oil can be used as a salad dressing.

Garlic—Rich in sulfur compounds, garlic ensures a steady rate of liver detoxification. These sulfur compounds also bind to heavy metals to escort them out of the body. Typically, people with high blood pressure often have low levels of sulfur compounds in their blood. Garlic also improves the liver's ability to lower cholesterol and blood pressure levels (when they are high). Scientists believe that garlic's compound prostaglandin A may be the effective ingredient that inhibits harmful liver enzymes and improves the way fats are metabolized in the liver.

As a bonus: garlic kills viruses, bacteria, and fungi and protects against heart disease too. Raw garlic is best, as some of the beneficial compounds break down with cooking. But cooked garlic is still helpful. Ideally, try to get at least one to two cloves of garlic daily. I've included many garlic-containing recipes at the back of this book to help you get started.

Leafy greens—As you learned earlier, salad greens are full of chlorophyll and enzymes that assist the liver with detoxification. Because chlorophyll is similar to red blood cells, it helps the body make healthy and clean blood. Because your liver is the main organ that filters the blood, chlorophyll helps in this regard. Leafy greens like spinach, spring mix, mustard greens, kale, collard, chard, and others are good sources of fiber and are nutritional powerhouses. Because the liver needs lots of nutrients to function properly, leafy greens are a serious asset. Obviously you can enjoy leafy greens as salads, or sauté kale, collard, and chard. You can add a handful of salad greens to a smoothie to ramp up its nutritional value. Check out the recipes in Chapter 10 to enjoy some liver-boosting green smoothies.

Lemons—The limonene found in lemon can boost your body's production of glutathione, a critical nutrient in liver detoxification that helps ensure toxins are neutralized. Lemons also contain over twenty anticancer compounds, so by enjoying fresh lemon in your water or a bit of grated rind in your baked goods (from organic lemons only), you'll help your liver eliminate cancer cells from your body before they can do damage.

Nuts and seeds—Consuming nuts can be as effective as cholesterol-lowering drugs to reduce high cholesterol levels, without the nasty side effects.[4] Walnuts, Brazil nuts, hazelnuts, almonds, pumpkin seeds, sunflower seeds, sesame seeds, and so forth are all great options. Be sure to choose raw, unsalted nuts and seeds, preferably those found in the refrigerator section of your local health food store.

Onions—Onions contain sulfur, which is required to increase enzyme activity that, in turn, boosts liver cleansing. Like garlic, onions also kill viruses, bacteria, and fungi.

Soy foods—Lecithin, found in soy foods, helps the liver metabolize fats and reduce cholesterol. Like eggs, it contains a substance called phosphatidylcholine and essential fatty acids that help keep liver cells healthy and prevent fatty deposits from building up in the liver. Lecithin also helps reduce high blood pressure by allowing the blood vessels to relax to allow better blood flow. Lecithin is naturally found in soy milk, tofu, and miso as well as organic eggs.

Turmeric—Not just for Indian curries anymore, this super-spice is potent medicine for the liver. It contains the highest known source of beta carotene, which helps protect the liver from free radical damage. It helps the liver metabolize fats by decreasing the fat storage rate in liver cells.[5] Enjoy turmeric in curries, soups, stews, or on its own in some water. For the latter, add one teaspoon of powdered turmeric to a cup of water, and drink—through a straw if possible, as turmeric can stain your teeth. It's liver-boosting properties are worth it, though, as turmeric is one of the best, if not the best, liver-boosting foods available.

Check out the recipes in Chapter 10 to discover many delicious foods, juices, and smoothies that contain the top twelve liver boosters. Be sure to try my Liver Jumpstart Juice on page 242.

The Supplements

In this section you'll discover the best nutrients and herbs that assist the liver with detoxification. You don't need to take all of them; just two or three is great. Reading the following section may give you some insight as to which ones might be best for you. Follow the dosage recommendations mentioned later in this section to maximize your chosen nutrients' liver-cleansing benefits.

Critical Nutrients for Liver Cleansing

There are many essential nutrients needed to ensure that liver detoxification can occur without a glitch. A single deficiency can impair proper liver cleansing and may result in seemingly unrelated but uncomfortable symptoms. So be sure you're taking a high-quality multivitamin and mineral. Keep reading to learn whether you might benefit from supplementing with one or more of the additional nutrients mentioned below. But, don't worry: the last thing I want is for you to be popping handfuls of supplements. You can choose two or three for your weekend.

Boost Your Liver with Vitamin C

Glutathione is one of the most important nutrients for maximum liver health and to feel great. It is a powerful ally for anyone looking to eliminate harmful toxins. Not only does it boost the liver's ability to detoxify harmful chemicals; it destroys free radicals all on its own. Although glutathione levels can become depleted over time or in the face of excessive toxins, it is fairly easy to boost the levels of the essential nutrient in your liver. Research shows that supplementing with at least 500mg of vitamin C daily boosts blood levels of glutathione by nearly 50 percent in healthy individuals.[6]

Supplement with 500 to 2000mg of vitamin C daily. Of course, there are many foods that can help boost glutathione levels as well, including asparagus, avocados, walnuts, cabbage, broccoli, Brussels sprouts, lemons, dill, and caraway seeds.

Taurine to Eliminate Excess Cholesterol
If you are suffering from high cholesterol or heart disease, then I recommend supplementing with the amino acid taurine because it not only helps with liver-related disorders but also helps the liver break down excess cholesterol. A typical cholesterol-lowering dose is 500mg twice daily.

Lecithin for a Fatty Liver
If you're trying to lower your cholesterol levels or to heal from a fatty liver, you may wish to supplement with lecithin. As you may recall, it is naturally found in eggs and soy foods, but sometimes the liver needs more lecithin than is found in these foods, particularly to heal a fatty liver. A typical fatty-liver healing dose is 4000mg of lecithin daily. It comes in capsules for convenience or granules that can be added to your liver-boosting smoothies.

More Liver-Boosting Nutritional Supplements
As you learned above, many nutrients, including vitamin C and S-adenosylmethionine (SAMe), are involved in liver detoxification. Of course there are many others, but most of these nutrients are found in a multivitamin and mineral supplement, so it doesn't need reiteration here. If you are suffering from fatigue, mood swings, or depression, take a 50 to 100mg B-complex supplement in addition to your multivitamin. You'll notice that some of the B-vitamins will be measured in micrograms, not milligrams— that's how some B vitamins are measured. For those vitamins, the dose would be 50 to 100mcg. If you're prone to PMS, you may wish to supplement with choline, vitamin B12, and folic acid, as these nutrients are needed to detoxify any excess hormones from the body. Because they are all B-complex vitamins, take a single 50 to 100mg B-complex supplement to avoid any deficiencies of these critical nutrients. If you've been on antibiotics several times in your life, you may benefit from supplementing your diet with vitamin B2, pantothenic acid (vitamin B5), and vitamin C, as

antibiotic drugs can deplete these nutrients in the liver. All of these nutrients, with the exception of vitamin C, are found in a good B-complex supplement.

Most multis contain fairly low amounts of vitamin C. If you've been under a lot of stress, are suffering from fatigue, or have taken antibiotics a few times in your life, you may benefit from extra vitamin C. An additional 1000mg is helpful taken at least a few hours away from other C vitamins you're taking.

If you're suffering from depression and want to boost your liver, supplementing with SAMe may be beneficial for you. Follow package instructions.

Select two nutrients and note them on the worksheet at the end of this chapter. (You can photocopy it for your use through the preparation stages and during the Love Your Liver Weekend detox.)

Herbal Liver Boosters

When it comes to strengthening the liver, herbs really shine. Most people don't realize how powerful herbs are, but pharmaceutical companies do. That's because many drugs are originally extracted from herbs. They become dangerous and potentially toxic once the pharmaceutical companies try to reproduce in a laboratory the substances nature created in a plant. As herbs, however, they are much safer and provide powerful medicine for the liver.

Although there are many great liver herbs, some of my favorite ones include milk thistle, dandelion root, globe artichoke, and turmeric. If you are pregnant or nursing, have a serious health condition, or are taking medication, consult a qualified health practitioner before using herbs.

Read the following herb descriptions. As you're reading them, pay attention to any that you feel particularly drawn to. Intuition goes a long way on a detox or health program, so I encourage you to trust your instincts. Of course, if you're taking any medications

or have any serious health conditions, you should consult a qualified health professional prior to taking any herbs. Choose one to
three herbs that feel right for you.

You can make the Love Your Liver Herbal Tea on page 244 if
you'd like. You can use capsules of milk thistle and turmeric (or
its extract, curcumin) if you prefer. The weekend detox is about
flexibility, so go with what feels right for you or what's available in
your local health food store, and then follow the suggested dosages
for each herb below.

Milk Thistle (Silybum marianum)

Milk thistle is commonly referred to as a "weed" because of its
prickly leaves and burrs that stick to clothing. Despite its seemingly pesky nature, milk thistle is one of the most powerful liver
medicines available. There are over one hundred studies that
demonstrate milk thistle's liver-protecting and regenerating properties, making it a proven choice for detoxifying and strengthening the liver. It contains a compound called silymarin that protects
the liver against cellular damage while also stimulating liver cells
to regenerate, enabling the liver to rebuild. If that wasn't enough,
milk thistle also prevents the depletion of the nutrient glutathione, which is essential for liver detoxification.

Silybin is another compound found in milk thistle that is believed to protect the genetic material within the liver cells while
reducing the occurrence of liver cancer.[7] Unlike other liver herbs,
milk thistle is best taken as a capsule or as an alcohol extract, as
the substances silymarin and silybin are not very water soluble,
meaning that a tea made from the plant won't have sufficient healing properties. Take three capsules daily containing at least 140mg
of silymarin each. Alternatively, take one teaspoon of the alcohol
extract three times daily unless you have ever been an alcoholic.

Dandelion Root (Taraxacum officinale)

Dandelion root is an herb in serious need of an image makeover.
Cursed by many gardeners and those in search of perfect lawns,
dandelion is frequently viewed as a pest and subsequently killed.

Ironically, however, most of the people killing this "weed" would experience greater health if they relied on the plant for medicine, as it has been proven in numerous studies to have beneficial healing effects on the liver. As far back as 1880, studies showed that dandelion is an effective treatment for hepatitis and swelling of the liver.[8] Another German study proved that dandelion root helped jaundice and reduced gallstones.[9] Newer research shows that dandelion root protects the liver against harmful toxins, such as carbon tetrachloride, which is used in some cleaning products and building materials.[10] The *Australian Journal of Medical Herbalism* cites research supporting the liver-regenerating properties of dandelion. Due to pesticides and pollutants, I don't recommend picking dandelion root from your lawn, though. You can take one to two teaspoons of dandelion root extract or supplement with 500 to 2000mg daily in capsules for two weeks to help cleanse your liver.

Globe Artichoke (Cynara scolymus)

Globe artichoke has effects similar to the herb milk thistle. It contains a group of compounds called caffeoylquinic acids, which have been shown in research to have powerful liver regenerative effects.[11] It has also been shown to be effective in treating serious liver conditions, including gallstones, liver damage, and liver insufficiency, but it is equally beneficial to strengthen the liver even if no serious liver conditions are present. It is typically found in capsule form, with doses ranging from 300 to 500mg. Consult the package of the product you choose to determine the exact dosage.

Turmeric (Curcuma longal)

You may recall turmeric from our discussion on the Top Twelve Liver-Boosting Foods. That's because turmeric is both a great food and herb. As one of the main spices used in Indian curries, it adds flavor and a bright yellow color to the foods with which it is cooked. It doesn't just taste great, however; it is also a liver cell regenerator and toxin eliminator. Its active ingredient, curcumin, is also an incredible anti-inflammatory that may help reduce liver inflammation. Research shows that curcumin increases two liver-supporting enzymes needed for healthy detoxification.

Turmeric and its active ingredient, curcumin, help reduce cholesterol levels while also reducing pain and inflammation throughout the body, so choose this herb if you are suffering from high cholesterol or any pain disorder. Curcumin comes in capsule form, which is probably the easiest way to get fairly high doses of this active ingredient, but you can also make a turmeric-honey mixture that you eat by the teaspoonful three times daily. Use equal parts of honey and turmeric, and store the mixture in a small jar. Of course, you can also cook with the dried or fresh turmeric root, but that is insufficient for most people to get adequate amounts of the therapeutic ingredients, so is best used in conjunction with one of the other forms. Check out some of the delicious recipes included in Chapter 10: Veggie Scramble on page 262 and Garbanzo Bean Squash Stew on page 265 both contain liver-healing turmeric.

Make a note about the herbs you have selected, and mark them on the worksheet found at the end of this chapter.

THE EXERCISE

The Crane Pose

As you now know, the liver is one of the main health-promoting organs. It filters your blood, helps burn fat, and even eliminates excess hormones and toxins to help maintain balance. In Chinese medicine an imbalanced liver can also be linked to digestive problems, headaches, depression, joint pain, fatigue, excess anger, and inflammation.

This qigong posture, which I call the Crane Pose, helps improve overall balance while also balancing the liver.

Begin by standing with your feet together. Extend your arms at shoulder height in front of you, keeping your palms facing forward. Take a deep breath.

Slowly move your arms to the sides, still at shoulder level. Gradually lift your knee with your toes pointing downward. Focus on expanding your chest. Exhale, and gradually lower your leg to the floor.

Repeat ten times, alternating the knee you lift each time. Be sure to practice this exercise very slowly and twice daily.

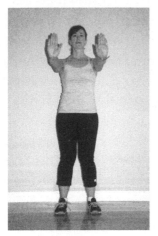
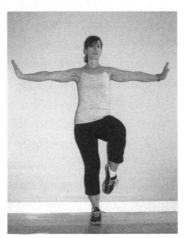

| Crane Pose 1 | Crane Pose 2 |

THE SPA TREATMENTS

The following are some wonderful therapies that can boost the effectiveness of your liver detoxification efforts. It isn't necessary to do all of them; rather, choose the one or ones that interest you most, and try to do them the specified number of times each day of the Love Your Liver Weekend. Of course, the more you choose, the better. But don't overwhelm yourself. If you think you can comfortably handle one, then just do that one. Remember that cleansing isn't a contest; it's an opportunity to do something wonderful for your body, mind, and spirit.

Easy Acupressure for Liver Detox and Healing

Acupressure, a powerful needle-free form of acupuncture, can help with liver detoxification. It is a simple, no-cost healing method that has survived the test of time for almost ten thousand years, probably due to its effectiveness.

Conducting acupressure is easy. Don't worry if you are unfamiliar with the points. With just a little practice, you'll have it mastered. Simply apply firm pressure to the points mentioned below (see the diagram that follows), and firmly hold each point for a minute or two. The points may be tender, but the tenderness usually subsides as you continue to hold the point. That's a sign that you've found the right point and that the acupressure is helping to disperse stagnant qi (pronounced "chee"), which means energy.

Start with the points Heart 8 and Liver 2 simultaneously, then move to Lung 8 and Liver 4 simultaneously. In other words, you'll hold two points at a time for this particular acupressure technique. Repeat on the opposite side of your body. See the diagram below to help you locate the points. The names of the points "Heart," "Liver," and "Lung" refer to the energy pathway on which the point sits and the corresponding organ to which it helps. So while you're working on this combination of points that is particularly good for the liver, it will also have benefits for the lungs and heart as well.

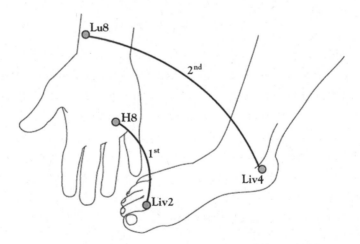

Heart 8 (H8) is located on the palm of the hand, about one inch below the webbing between the little finger and ring finger.

Liver 2 (Liv2) is located on the top of the foot where the big toe and the second toe meet.

Then:

Lung 8 (Lu8) is located on the inside of the arm, on the thumb side, about one inch higher than the wrist crease.

Liver 4 (Liv4) is located on the front of the ankle bone on the inside of the leg.

Liver-Healing Aromatherapy Compress

It may be hard to imagine that a cloth compress with carefully selected essential oils could have any effect on your liver, but it can. Your skin is your body's largest detoxification organ, but it also absorbs directly into your blood anything you put on it. That spells huge liver-healing benefits if you apply an aromatherapy compress over your liver.

Your liver is situated just below your lower right ribs on the front of your body. By placing a compress over the liver, oils are absorbed directly into the blood that feeds this organ, helping it to cleanse.

To experience the liver-healing aromatherapy compress you'll need:

Three layers of unbleached or uncolored cotton flannel (approximately twelve inches by six inches)

One-half to one cup of castor oil (available in most health food stores)

One or two essential oils: peppermint (menthe piperita), lemon (citrus limon), celery (apium graveolens), or carrot (daucus carota)*

A dry cloth to place between the cotton flannel and the hot water bottle

Hot water bottle or electric heating pad

---

*You can still experience this spa treatment if you don't have the essential oils—just use the castor oil.

Stack the three layers of cotton flannel on top of each other. On the top layer pour the castor oil so it is saturated but not dripping. Add your selected aromatherapy oils. Place the compress over the liver area.

Place a dry cloth over the flannel sheets. Top with the water bottle or electric heating pad. Lay back and relax for thirty to sixty minutes.

Use this therapy all three days of the Love Your Liver Weekend.

THE WEEKEND

You've learned a lot about the liver, what it does, the health conditions with which it is linked, and the foods, nutrients, herbs, exercise, and therapies that give it a boost. Don't worry if it seems a bit overwhelming right now—we'll be putting it all together here.

I've outlined a step-by-step approach to the Love Your Liver Weekend detox below. Of course, you can substitute other foods. I've listed some excellent liver-boosting recipes to help you get started. There's no need to eat or drink all of the items suggested. If you have the Super-Detoxifying Green Tea Lemonade midmorning, you don't need to drink the Love Your Liver Herbal Tea too. Try to maintain a lot of variety: if you have the Citrus Boost juice at lunch, have the herbal tea later. If you snack on walnuts midmorning, try an avocado salad midafternoon.

The Love Your Liver Weekend detox is designed to be flexible and individualized so you'll get the best results.

Here's what your three-day weekend will look like:

Days one to three:

Upon rising—Drink a large glass of water (two cups) with the fresh juice of one lemon. Add a few drops of liquid stevia if you prefer a sweeter-tasting beverage. Wait twenty minutes before eating.

Breakfast—Explore the breakfast options in the recipe section of this book. Be sure to include some of the liver-boosting foods mentioned above. Some good options include Liver Jumpstart Juice (page 242), Veggie Scramble (page 262), a soft-boiled egg with Lemon-Garlic Greens (page 252), or a bowl of brown rice topped with warm almond milk.

Multivitamin

Optional nutrients

Herb (first dose of selected herbs) or a cup of Love Your Liver Herbal Tea (page 244).

Midmorning—Large glass of water (with lemon if desired) or a cup of Love Your Liver Herbal Tea (page 244) or Super-Detoxifying Green Tea Lemonade (page 243).

Snack, such as an apple, raw unsalted walnuts, a Health-Building Gourmet Salad topped with avocado (page 254), or celery sticks with almond butter or Herbes de Provence Cashew Cheese (page 250)

Exercise—the crane pose

Easy acupressure for liver detox

Lunch—Weekend Wonder Detox Signature Salad (page 258) or other large detoxifying salad topped with some of Dr. Michelle's Top Twelve Liver-Boosting Foods

Liver Jumpstart Juice (page 242), Honey-Turmeric Tea (page 247), or Love Your Liver Herbal Tea (page 244)

Vitamin C

Optional nutrients

Herb (second dose of selected herbs, not required if you drank Love Your Liver Herbal Tea)

Midafternoon—Large glass of water (with lemon if desired) or a cup of Love Your Liver Herbal Tea (page 244) or Citrus Boost (page 241)

Snack, such as apple with almond butter, raw unsalted walnuts, an apple, or celery sticks with almond butter or Herbes de Provence Cashew Cheese (page 250)

Exercise—the crane pose

Easy acupressure for liver detox

Dinner—Spicy, Rice-y Detox Soup (page 260) with Lemon-Garlic Greens (page 252) or Roasted Red Pepper Chickpea Mash (page 263) with Cucumber-Mint Salad or Ginger Chili Quinoa (page 264)

Fresh cup of Liver Jumpstart Juice (page 242), Love Your Liver Herbal Tea (page 244), or Honey-Turmeric Tea (page 247)

Herb (third dose of selected herb, not required if you drank Love Your Liver Herbal Tea)

After dinner—Large glass of water (with lemon if desired) or a cup of Love Your Liver Herbal Tea (page 244) or Citrus Boost (page 241)

Liver-healing aromatherapy compress

Before bed—Take some quiet time to turn off the television. Find a quiet place to sit, close your eyes, and take some deep breaths.

Write in Love Your Liver Weekend Detox Journal (at the end of this chapter)

CONCLUDING THE LOVE YOUR LIVER WEEKEND

Congratulations! You just did something wonderful to boost the health of your liver and your whole body. Completing the Love Your Liver Weekend is something you should feel proud of.

After the Love Your Liver Weekend you may wish to keep incorporating foods, nutrients, herbs, exercises, or spa treatments into your day-to-day life. I encourage you to do so. Your liver is such an important organ; nurturing it through these healthy options can make a huge difference to your health.

Alternatively, you may wish to do the Love Your Liver Weekend every weekend for a month or one weekend out of every month. The choice is yours. You know your lifestyle and schedule best, so choose the option that works best for you.

If you continue to follow the Love Your Liver Weekend for longer periods, just take one week off from any herbs you're using after every three weeks.

And be sure to try some of the other health-building weekend detoxes I've included throughout *Weekend Wonder Detox*. If you're still feeling sluggish or suffering from any types of joint or muscle pain, you may want to opt for the Lymphomania Weekend next.

THE WORKSHEETS

The Grocery List

For easy Love Your Liver Weekend prep, print this list and take it with you when you go to your local health food and grocery stores. Remember that not all of the items are essential; purchase only the foods, nutrients, herbs, and items for the spa treatments you've selected.

Foods

Here are the liver-boosting foods you'll need. Also, make sure your pantry is stocked with the essential items you learned about in Chapter 2 for any recipes you select.

— lemons (for morning lemon water)
Other liver-boosting foods
— avocado
— beets
— dandelion greens
— eggs
— flax seeds or flax seed oil
— garlic
— leafy greens
— lemons (in addition to the morning lemon water)
— nuts and seeds
— onions
— soy foods
— turmeric

Nutritional Supplements
— multivitamin and mineral (essential)
— vitamin C (essential)
— B-complex (optional)
— amino acid complex (optional)
— taurine (optional)

— lecithin (optional)

— SAMe (optional)

Herbs

Choose one to three of the following herbs:

— milk thistle

— dandelion root

— globe artichoke

— turmeric

Optional Items if You Selected the
Liver-Healing Aromatherapy Compress

— unbleached cotton flannel (enough for three layers of twelve inches by six inches)

— castor oil

— one or two of the following pure essential oils: peppermint (mentha piperita), lemon (citrus limon), celery (apium graveolens), or carrot (daucus carota)

— dry cloth

— hot water bottle or electric heating pad

The Love Your Liver Weekend Detox Journal

You may wish to print off a copy of the journal page to make it easier to complete.

Energy: Rate your energy (from 0 to 10, with 0 meaning complete exhaustion, and 10 meaning abundant energy). Before the detox _____ After the detox _____

Pain: Rate your pain levels (from 0 to 10, with 0 meaning none, and 10 meaning unbearable, constant pain). Before the detox _____ After the detox _____

Mood: Rate your mood (from 0 to 10, with 0 meaning extremely moody, depressed, angry, or irritable, and 10 meaning extremely happy). Before the detox _____ After the detox _____

Weight: Before the detox _____ After the detox _____

Checklist of Liver-Boosting Foods Consumed

Try to eat at least five a day. Check the ones you eat each day.

	Day 1	Day 2	Day 3
avocado	_____	_____	_____
beets	_____	_____	_____
dandelion greens	_____	_____	_____
eggs	_____	_____	_____
flax seeds or flax seed oil	_____	_____	_____
garlic	_____	_____	_____
leafy greens	_____	_____	_____
lemons	_____	_____	_____
nuts and seeds	_____	_____	_____
onions	_____	_____	_____
soy foods	_____	_____	_____
turmeric	_____	_____	_____

Selected Nutrients

Be sure to take the multivitamin and vitamin C each day. Write down any additional nutrients you've opted to take throughout the detox. Remember, you don't need to take all of them. Check off each day you take them.

	Day 1	Day 2	Day 3
multivitamin and mineral	_____	_____	_____
vitamin C	_____	_____	_____
B-complex	_____	_____	_____

continues

Selected Nutrients *continued*

	Day 1	Day 2	Day 3
amino acid complex	_____	_____	_____
taurine	_____	_____	_____
lecithin	_____	_____	_____
SAMe	_____	_____	_____

Selected Herbs

Indicate the one to three herbs you've selected to take throughout the detox. Check off each day you take them. Most herbs need to be taken three times daily.

	Day 1	Day 2	Day 3
milk thistle	_____	_____	_____
dandelion root	_____	_____	_____
globe artichoke	_____	_____	_____
turmeric	_____	_____	_____

Exercise

Check off each time you complete the Crane Pose. Make sure to do it every day.

	Day 1	Day 2	Day 3
The Crane Pose	_____	_____	_____

Selected Spa Treatment(s)

Check off each time you complete the liver-boosting spa treatments. It's not necessary to do both of them, but whichever one(s) you choose, make sure you do it every day.

	Day 1	Day 2	Day 3
acupressure	——	——	——
aromatherapy compress	——	——	——

Observations and Thoughts

Day 1: _____

_____

_____

_____

Day 2: _____

_____

_____

_____

Day 3: _____

_____

_____

_____

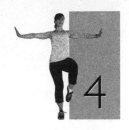

THE LYMPHOMANIA WEEKEND

BENEFITS OF DETOXIFYING YOUR LYMPHATIC SYSTEM

- Pain reduction
- Weight loss
- Less bloating
- Reduced eye puffiness

The lymphatic system is one of the most important cleansing and healing systems in your body. It is frequently the difference between poor and good health.

Harvey Diamond, natural health pioneer and author of *Fit for Life*, the world's best-selling health book author of all time, describes a healthy lymphatic system as the "number one factor in achieving good health."[1] Yet few doctors ever mention that your lymphatic system is overloaded when you are experiencing health problems.

WHAT IS THE LYMPHATIC SYSTEM, AND WHY SHOULD I DETOXIFY IT?

The lymphatic system is a complex network of fluid-filled nodes, glands, and tubes that bathe our cells and that carry the body's

NELLY'S FIBROMYALGIA PAIN VANISHES

Nelly, a petite sixty-four-year-old woman, came to see me complaining of fibromyalgia pain that she had been suffering from for over a decade. While she was still working as an information technology professional she informed me that it was getting harder and harder to maintain her duties due to the pain. When I asked her to rate the pain from zero to ten, with ten being the worst pain she had ever felt, Nelly rated the pain as a ten, so I knew she was struggling with it. Like many people suffering from pain disorders, Nelly no longer had much capacity for hobbies, exercise, or other activities—the pain was definitely affecting the quality of her life.

I know from experience that most people with fibromyalgia also suffer from lymphatic congestion. So I immediately asked her to follow the Lymphomania Weekend Cleanse. She agreed wholeheartedly.

Fibromyalgia is such a complex and chronic condition that I realized Nelly might need longer than three days to experience the improvement she hoped for. But I asked her to start with three days and to report back to me after that so we could decide on the next steps for her.

She contacted me three days later to report that days one and two had been difficult for her to make the dietary changes and to figure out what she could and could not eat. By day three her pain level had already dropped. She rated it a seven but still wasn't convinced the lymph cleanse was responsible. Nonetheless, she agreed to keep going with the cleanse for a week, at which point she rated the pain a five. She told me she wanted to continue to see whether she could reduce the pain even further. By this point she was convinced of the power of the Lymphomania Cleanse.

Nelly came back to see me four weeks after her initial appointment. She was "bouncing off the walls" with excitement and energy. She exclaimed, "I can't believe how good I feel. I'm so much better." When I asked her to rate her pain levels she said, "No, no, you don't understand. I don't have ANY pain anymore." She added, "I can't believe I suffered for thirteen years when the solution was so simple." She signed up for a co-ed bike race, beating men and women half her age. Nelly had a new lease on life. Now when the pain creeps up, Nelly knows it's time for a Lymphomania Weekend.

"sewage" away from the tissues and then neutralize it. It also includes the spleen, thymus, and tonsils, all of which work together to clean up your bodily cells and tissues and to remove harmful toxins before they can contribute to pain and illness.

The lymphatic system handles toxins that enter your body from external sources (exotoxins), such as foods or air pollution, but also handles internally produced toxins (endotoxins) that are the result of normal metabolic processes in your body. One example is inflammation in the body. The lymph system helps carry the waste products of inflammation to your blood to be eliminated.

Lymph fluid, a clear, slightly yellowish fluid, enters the bloodstream at the veins near your heart. Once toxins have been swept up in the lymph system and dumped into the bloodstream, the kidneys take over to filter the blood of any toxins.

In an interview Ann Louise Gittleman, PhD, author of *The Fat Flush*, cites a study in which researchers found that 80 percent of overweight women have sluggish lymphatic systems.[2] Getting them flowing smoothly is the key to easy weight loss and improved feelings of well-being.

Another study by Elisabeth Dancey, MD, author of *The Cellulite Solution*, found that women with cellulite showed lymphatic system deficiencies.[3] When you thoroughly cleanse your lymphatic system you will see cellulite diminish.

There is three times more lymph fluid in the body than blood, yet the lymphatic system has no organ like a heart to help pump it. Instead, the lymph system relies on deep breathing, exercise, and massage to flow effectively. By boosting the health of your lymphatic system you are also purifying your blood, as the blood is filtered through the largest mass of lymph tissue, the spleen. The spleen fights infection and destroys worn-out red blood cells in the body. Located just left of the stomach, the spleen aids your overall immunity against infection.

During Weekend Wonder Detox you will begin to improve the flow of the lymphatic system using foods, nutrients, herbs, and natural spa treatments. The Lymphomania and Love Your Liver

Weekends go hand in hand, so you may wish to do the latter detox on another weekend after you've completed the Lymphomania weekend. This will further aid your lymphatic system because the liver is primarily responsible for producing lymph fluid.

SIGNS OF A
STRESSED-OUT LYMPHATIC SYSTEM

You don't have to be diagnosed with a serious health condition like fibromyalgia or another pain disorder to have signs of a stressed-out lymphatic system. Because everyone's body is different, you might have one symptom, or you could have many signs of lymph congestion.

SIGNS YOU WOULD BENEFIT FROM A LYMPHOMANIA WEEKEND	
overweight or obesity	lupus
cellulite	other chronic immune system disorder
fatty deposits	
aches and pains	bloating or edema of your bodily tissues
fibromyalgia (diagnosed by a doctor)	
	lumps or growths on your body
chronic fatigue syndrome (diagnosed by a doctor)	abdominal bloating
	eye puffiness
multiple sclerosis	

The lymphatic system is linked with many different symptoms and conditions because it is such an integral part of the body's toxin-removal systems. Your body relies on the lymphatic system to remove internally generated toxins from its many life-essential biochemical activities and from metabolizing food. And the onslaught of chemicals from our environment can easily overwhelm this critical system.

THE DIET

In addition to the recommendations outlined in Chapter 2, it is important to abide by the following recommendations. You may notice that some of the advice repeats that of Chapter 2, but I think it is important for you to understand some of the suggestions in the context of the lymphatic system.

1. **Drink plenty of water.** Although I stated this earlier, it is important to consider this recommendation in the context of the lymphatic system. Without adequate water, lymph fluid cannot flow properly. To help ensure my cells readily absorb the water, I frequently add some fresh lemon juice, but that is up to you while following the Lymphomania Weekend.

2. **Avoid processed, packaged, and prepared foods.** It is critical to realize that food additives, preservatives, colors, artificial sweeteners, and harmful fats clog the lymphatic system, adding work to its already large load. Eliminating them from your diet gives the lymphatic system time to catch up on its cleansing tasks.

3. **Forget the soda, trash the neon-colored sports drinks, and drop the fruit "juices"** that are more sugar than fruit. These sugar-, color-, and preservative-laden beverages add to the already overburdened workload your lymph system must handle.

4. **Eliminate all dairy and wheat products for the weekend.** Many people have hidden sensitivities to these foods that result in bloating and sluggish tissues. By eliminating all sources of these foods you'll give your body a short break. You may also wish to forego them after the detox is finished. Obviously cheese, milk, butter, ice cream, and cream are dairy products, but don't forget the foods that contain them, such as breads, buns, desserts, and cookies. Wheat is found in most prepared, processed, and packaged foods, but, because you're already avoiding these foods, that will help a lot.

5. **Eat more raw fruit on an empty stomach.** The enzymes and acids in fruit are powerful lymph cleansers. Eat them on an empty stomach for best digestion and maximum lymph-cleansing

benefits. Most fruits are digested within thirty minutes or so and quickly help you feel better.

6. **Eat plenty of green vegetables** to get adequate chlorophyll to help purify your blood and lymph.

7. **Eat raw, unsalted nuts and seeds** to power up your lymph with adequate fatty acids. Choose from walnuts, almonds, hazelnuts, macadamias, Brazil nuts, flax seeds, sunflower seeds, and pumpkin seeds.

Dr. Michelle's Top Six Lymph-Boosting Foods

If you want to rev up your lymphatic system, you will want to include some of the best lymph superfoods. Here are some of my favorites.

Cranberries and cranberry juice—Flavonoids, malic acid, citric acid, quinic acid, and enzymes (only in raw cranberries and raw cranberry juice, not in pasteurized bottled cranberry juice) in cranberries and cranberry juice help to emulsify stubborn fat in the lymphatic system, allowing the body to break it down for elimination. If you're drinking cranberry juice, be sure to drink only pure, cranberry juice, free of added sweeteners. Dilute it about 4:1 water to cranberry juice. I'm not talking about the sweetened variety that has almost no juice and more closely resembles cranberry cocktail; I'm talking about 100 percent pure, unsweetened cranberry juice. If you need it to taste a bit sweeter, either add a few drops of stevia or a tiny splash of organic apple juice. Also avoid apple juice with preservatives.

Leafy greens—Chlorophyll doesn't just give leafy greens their dark green color; it's also a superb lymphatic cleanser. Leafy greens are packed with many other critical vitamins and minerals to help boost your lymph cleansing efforts. You'll want to eat lots of these nutritional powerhouse foods during this weekend, including salad greens (mixed mesclun, Romaine lettuce, leaf lettuce, Boston lettuce, or another type of salad mix), kale, collards, bok choy, spinach, or watercress.

Flax seeds and flax seed oil—Flax seeds and flax seed oil help reduce inflammation within the lymph system so the body can eliminate toxins. Because the delicate Omega 3s go rancid easily, all flax seeds and oil should be kept refrigerated, including in the store where you purchase them. It's also best to buy flax seeds whole and then grind your own in a coffee grinder for each use. To use the seeds, add them to smoothies or on top of toast, dips, bread, or crudité and almond butter. Top cooked vegetables or salads with a bit of flax oil. Use flax oil in homemade salad dressing recipes (see the Recipes section for ideas).

Nuts and seeds—Foods high in essential fatty acids are critical to ensure a properly functioning lymph system. Some of these foods include fresh, raw walnuts, almonds, hazelnuts, macadamias, Brazil nuts, and other types of nuts, sunflower seeds, flax seeds (they're important enough to warrant a second mention!), pumpkin seeds, avocadoes, and cold-pressed nut oils.

Sprouts—Sprouts are some of the healthiest lymph-cleansing foods you can eat. That's because the nutritional count skyrockets when seeds are soaked and sprouted. The energy contained in the seed, grain, nut, or legume is ignited and its nutrients unlocked, providing plenty of health benefits and energy. Research shows that during the sprouting process mung bean sprouts (or just bean sprouts, as they are often called) increase in vitamin B1 by up to 285 percent, vitamin B2 by up to 515 percent, and niacin by up to 256 percent. Essential fatty acids also increase during the sprouting process.

Here are some easy ways to get plenty of sprouts into your diet: add a handful to your favorite salad, throw a large handful of mung bean sprouts into your favorite noodle dish or stir-fry after you've removed it from the heat and are ready to serve it, add alfalfa or clover sprouts to a sandwich or wrap, spice up a salad or sandwich with mustard or radish sprouts, or make sprouts the focal point of your meal by using mung bean, alfalfa, clover, or other mild sprouts as the base for a delicious salad topped with raw or roasted veggies. Simply add grated or julienned (cut into matchsticks) vegetables like red or green peppers, carrots, celery, cucumbers, or any others you prefer.

THE SUPPLEMENTS

In this section you'll discover the best nutrients and herbs that assist the lymphatic system with detoxification. You don't need to take all of them; just two or three is great. Reading the following section may give you some insight into which ones might be best for you. Follow the dosage recommendations mentioned later in this section to maximize the cleansing benefits of your chosen nutrients.

Critical Nutrients for Lymph Cleansing

There are many essential nutrients needed to ensure that the lymphatic system can detoxify properly. Beta carotene and vitamin A neutralize damaging free radicals and support lymph tissue in escorting toxins out. The minerals iron, selenium, and zinc are needed to make sufficient white blood cells, which circulate in the lymph system and kill harmful microbes. All of these nutrients can be obtained in a single high-quality multivitamin, which was recommended in Chapter 2. Follow package instructions. A single deficiency can impair proper cleansing and may result in seemingly unrelated but uncomfortable symptoms. So be sure you're taking a high-quality multivitamin and mineral.

Keep reading to learn whether you might benefit from supplementing with one or more of the additional nutrients mentioned below. But don't worry: I don't want you taking many supplements for the weekend detox.

Vitamin C

Vitamin C assists in the proper flow of lymph. It basically functions by helping to scrub toxins out of your body's cells so they can be eliminated. Vitamin C is also important for tissue repair. Take

2000mg of vitamin C twice daily in divided doses to ensure proper absorption.

Protease to Power Up Your Lymph

Protease is a category of enzymes that break down proteins. It works to clean up the lymph and keep it moving at a sufficient pace by breaking down toxins that have a protein outer membrane, which many toxins do, particularly viruses, bacteria, cancer cells, and inflammation. Protease can be taken as a single supplement or as part of a full-spectrum digestive enzyme supplement. Either way, it needs to be taken on an empty stomach, away from food, to work on the lymphatic system. Take three tablets or capsules three times daily at least thirty minutes before eating or one hour after eating. Choose a brand that guarantees no genetically modified organisms (GMOs) are used, as many enzymes are sourced from genetically modified ingredients.

Herbal Lymph System Boosters

Although there are many great lymph-boosting herbs, some of my favorite ones include Echinacea, astragalus, cleavers, and wild indigo root. If you are pregnant or nursing, have a serious health condition, or are taking medication, consult a qualified health practitioner before using herbs.

Don't worry: you don't need to purchase all of the lymph-strengthening herbs; one to three is sufficient. I've included extra ones, should you have difficulty finding any of the herbs in stores. Of course, you don't need to pick them yourself, as most health food stores have them in dried, capsule, or tincture (alcohol-extract) form.

Although alcohol extracts are great, avoid using alcohol extract if you have ever been an alcoholic or if you are diabetic.

Read the following herb descriptions. As you're reading them, pay attention to any that you feel particularly drawn to. Intuition goes a long way on a detox or health program, so I encourage you to trust your instincts. Of course, if you're taking any medications or have any serious health conditions, you should consult a qualified health professional prior to taking any herbs. Choose one to three herbs that feel right for you.

You can make the Lymphomania Herbal Tea on page 245 if you'd like. If you wish to drink this herb tea instead of taking tinctures or herbal supplements, that's fine. In that case drink one cup of the tea three times daily. As with all of the detoxes, the Lymphomania Weekend is about flexibility, so go with what feels right for you or what's available in your local health food store, and then follow the suggested dosages for each herb below.

Echinacea (Echinacea, various species)

Most people have heard of echinacea as a cold or flu remedy or as an herbal immune-boosting remedy, but it is also a powerful lymphatic system cleanser. Combined with astragalus, echinacea helps to lessen congestion and swelling and get the lymph fluid moving better. Make a decoction by using two teaspoons of dried herb per cup of water, bring to a boil, and then reduce to a simmer for fifteen minutes. Drink one cup, or one teaspoon of tincture, three times per day.

Astragalus (Astragalus, various species)

Astragalus is an excellent lymphatic system cleanser, particularly in combination with echinacea. Like the former herb, it also helps to alleviate congestion and swelling in the body. Astragalus is primarily available as a tincture or in capsule or tablet form. Take one teaspoon of tincture, three times per day.

Cleavers (Galium aparine, also known as goosegrass or grip grass)

Cleavers is a natural anti-inflammatory remedy that also enhances all functions of the lymphatic system. It is, therefore, an excellent herb for lymph cleansing and to reduce swelling in various parts of the lymph system, such as swollen glands or tonsils. Use two to three teaspoons of the dried herb per cup of boiled water to make cleavers tea. Drink one cup three times daily. You can use one tea-spoon of alcohol extract of cleavers (tincture) three times daily if you prefer. Diabetics should avoid using cleavers.

Wild Indigo Root (Baptisia tinctoria)

Wild indigo root kills bacteria and viruses in the body while break-ing down excess mucous and improving lymph flow. It cleans up the lymphatic system and is a great choice if you are also prone to sinus or nasal congestion. It also reduces swelling in the glands, larynx, pharynx, and tonsils. It works especially well when com-bined with echinacea or cleavers. Make a decoction-type of tea by boiling one-third teaspoon of the dried root per cup of water in a pot. Bring to a boil, and then cover and reduce the heat to allow to simmer for one hour. Drink one cup of this extraction three times daily. Alternatively, use one-half teaspoon of alcohol tincture, available in many health food stores, three times daily.

Consult an herbalist or natural medicine specialist before taking herbs with any medications or if you suffer from a serious health condition. Avoid using herbs while pregnant or lactating, and avoid long-term use of any herb without first consulting a qualified professional.

THE EXERCISE

Rebounding

Exercise is needed to ensure the lymphatic system flows prop-erly. The best kind of lymph-boosting exercise is rebounding on a minitrampoline, as this dramatically improves lymph flow but is also great for boosting circulation and is a superb low-impact form of exercise that could be used with any of the detoxes. Rebounders are about three feet in diameter, so they can easily be stored in a closet or in the corner of a living room. It's basically jumping on a minitrampoline. It's easy to rebound while you are watching tele-vision, so even couch potatoes can handle this form of exercise.

Rebounders are inexpensive (usually around $50) and available in most department and sports stores. Ideally, rebound for at least ten minutes, but twenty is preferable. Rebound all three days of your weekend detox to help keep lymph toxins moving through and out of your body.

If you can't afford one, aerobic exercise of any kind will help get the lymphatic system moving better. Do at least twenty minutes of aerobic activity like running, jogging, brisk walking, elliptical training, or StairMaster daily for each day of the weekend.

THE SPA TREATMENTS

Lymph-Booster Massage

Vigorous massage of areas of the body known as the "neurolymphatic points" can help get toxins moving, improve circulation, and even boost your energy. These points act like circuit breakers or switches in the circulation of energy to the lymphatic system. Sometimes when there is stagnation through lack of movement or excess toxic buildup the points become overloaded and stop supplying sufficient energy to the lymphatic system to eliminate the toxins.

Studies show that virtually any type of massage can push up to 78 percent of stagnant lymph back into circulation.[4] Massage frees trapped toxins, and neurolymphatic massage is particularly good at freeing these toxins.

I've included a diagram of the neurolymphatic massage points to help you locate them. Don't worry about precision; you'll know you found them because many neurolymphatic points feel tender. That's typically a sign of stagnation and indicates the need to massage these points. Massage as many of the points as you can. You may need a partner to reach some of the points on the back. There is no specific order to the points—just follow the diagram and try to rub all of them.

You can perform this massage clothed, and it can take place almost anywhere. Just take three to five minutes daily to massage

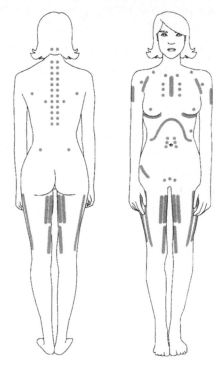

Figure 4.1

the points in Figure 4.1. Ideally, repeat this procedure at least twice daily on all three days of your Lymphomania Weekend. Use firm, deep pressure that is still manageable. This is not a muscle strength contest, so don't overdo and cause bruising. You don't have to worry about getting all the points accurate. Just rub the general area for a few seconds each. You'll know you've found the right points if they are tender. It looks more complicated than it is, but just do your best to rub as many of the points as you can. The whole thing shouldn't take more than a few minutes and will tremendously boost lymph circulation as well as blood circulation.

Pay particular attention to the tender points. The tenderness will usually decrease as you massage them.

Most people not only experience an increase of energy but often a reduction in pain as well simply by massaging the neurolymphatic points. Rub your neurolymphatic points two or three times daily while following the Lymphomania Weekeend. Of course, you can continue to rub these points after the weekend is over or any time you need a boost of energy or a decrease in pain.

Dry Skin Brushing

Dry skin brush before showering. Use a natural bristle brush (brushes are readily available everywhere, from online to chain stores). If you can't find one, just use a dry, fairly rough washcloth. Use a firm pressure, but we're not trying to inflict pain or damage your skin. Brush your dry skin in circular motions upward from the feet to the torso and from the fingers to the chest. You want to work in the same direction as your lymph flows—toward the heart.

So start with the tops of your feet (no need to do the bottoms), and in circular motions brush up the front of your leg toward your hips, then start back at the foot and brush up the outside of your leg toward your hips, then brush from your foot up the inside of your leg, and finally the back of your leg. Repeat on the other leg. Avoid dry brushing the genitals and the breast region.

Then dry brush your torso. First dry brush up the front of your abdomen toward the heart, then brush up each side of the abdomen and the back toward your heart, always in circular motions and always toward the heart.

Then dry brush the palm of your hand in circles upward along the inside of your arm toward your armpit. Return to the hand, and dry brush the top of the hand and the outside of your arm toward your shoulder. Then return to the hand, and dry brush each side of your arm toward your shoulder. Repeat on the other arm. Finally, dry brush over the collarbone area from the armpit toward the heart. Repeat on the other side.

It sounds like a lot, but, once you get the hang of it, the whole process takes only a minute or two in the morning before you shower. Of course, you should also avoid dry brushing any open wounds and skin infections.

Most people notice that they start to feel more energized after a few days of following this procedure. Circulation improves, and even skin conditions begin to improve. Over time dry skin brushing can also help the body eliminate excess bloating in the tissues by getting the lymphatic system moving more effectively. Dry skin brush in the morning before showering for all three days on the Lymphomania Weekend. Of course, you can continue this excellent habit after the three days are over if you'd like. I've had clients enjoy the feel of dry skin brushing so much that they continue it for years. It's up to you.

Optional: after showering, while your skin is still damp, apply the Lymphomania Massage Oil (you'll find the recipe in the Recipe section at the back of this book). It contains essential oils like geranium, juniper, and black pepper that stimulate the lymphatic system through massage and improve the flow of lymph, thereby helping your body eliminate toxins.

THE WEEKEND

You're now quite familiar with the lymphatic system, the foods that strengthen it, and the nutrients, herbs, exercises, and spa treatments that give it a boost. If it feels a bit overwhelming, don't worry: we'll be putting it all together here.

I've outlined a step-by-step approach to the Lymphomania Weekend detox below. Of course, you can substitute other foods. I've listed some excellent lymphatic system cleansing recipes to help you get started. But you don't need to eat or drink these specific foods if others interest you more. Just be sure to eat plenty of the Top Lymph-Boosting Foods outlined above.

There are lots of customization options. I've done that intentionally to ensure you have a personalized plan that fits your health needs, budget, and schedule. Here's what your three-day weekend will look like.

Days one to three:

Upon rising—Drink a large glass of water (two cups) with fresh juice of one-half lemon or Lymphomania Herbal Tea (page

245) or Cranberry Green Tea Lemonade (page 243). Add a few drops of liquid stevia if you prefer a sweeter-tasting beverage. Wait twenty minutes before eating.

Dry skin brush

Breakfast—Be sure to include some of the lymph-cleansing foods mentioned above. Some good options include Cranberry Pear Juice (page 242), Chia Breakfast Tapioca with ground flax seeds sprinkled on top (page 266), a soft-boiled egg with Lemon-Garlic Greens (page 252), or cooked brown rice with almond milk.

Multivitamin

Optional nutrients

Herb (first dose of selected herbs)

Midmorning—Large glass of water (with lemon if desired), a cup of Lymphomania Herbal Tea (page 245), or Super-Detoxifying Green Tea Lemonade (page 243)

Snack, such as an apple with almond butter, raw, unsalted walnuts, a bowl of berries or Heirloom Tomato and Basil Salad (page 257), or celery sticks with almond butter or Herbes de Provence Cashew Cheese (page 250)

Exercise—rebounding

Lymph-booster massage

Lunch—Weekend Wonder Detox Signature Salad (page 258) or other large detoxifying salad with added sprouts (mung, alfalfa, clover, etc.)

Celery Cucumber Juice (page 240), Cranberry Green Tea Lemonade (page 243), or Honey-Turmeric Tea (page 247)

Vitamin C

Optional nutrients

Herb (second dose of selected herbs)

Midafternoon—Large glass of water (with lemon if desired), a cup of Lymphomania Herbal Tea (page 245), or Carrot Celery Juice (page 240) with Cucumber-Mint Salad (page 258)

Snack, such as grapefruit, apple, raw, unsalted walnuts, Cucumber-Mint Salad (page 258), or an apple with almond butter

Exercise—rebounding

Dinner—Thai Coconut Vegetable Soup (page 261) or Lentil Bowl (page 263) and Chili Lime Green Beans (page 252)

Cucumber-Mint Refresh (page 240) and Honey-Turmeric Tea (page 247)

Herb (third dose of selected herb)

After dinner—Large glass of water (with lemon if desired), a cup of Lymphomania Herbal Tea (page 245), or Watermelon Ice (page 241)

Before bed—Take some quiet time to turn off the television. Find a quiet place to sit, close your eyes, and take some deep breaths.

Write in the Lymphomania Weekend Detox Journal (at the end of this chapter).

CONCLUDING THE LYMPHOMANIA WEEKEND

If lymph is stagnant, there is an increased toxic load in the body. This can affect memory and mental function and contribute to inflammation, pain, and bloating. It can result in cellulite, fatty deposits, and disorders like fibromyalgia and chronic fatigue syndrome, among others. Getting lymph moving freely is the key to better health, reduced pain, and even more energy. Congratulations on taking a huge step toward better health by completing the Lymphomania Weekend.

After the Lymphomania Weekend you may wish to keep incorporating foods, nutrients, herbs, exercises, or spa treatments into your day-to-day life. I encourage you to do so. Your lymphatic system is critical to great health, so regular care and maintenance through the simple rebounding, massage, skin brushing, and enjoying lymph-boosting foods, nutrients, and herbs can make a huge difference to your health.

Alternatively, you may wish to do the Lymphomania Weekend every weekend for a month or one weekend out of every month.

The choice is yours. You know your lifestyle and schedule best. Choose the option that works best for you.

If you continue to follow the Lymphomania Weekend for longer periods, every three weeks just take one week off from any herbs you're using.

And don't forget to try some of the other health-building weekend detoxes I've included throughout *Weekend Wonder Detox*. Your body will love you for it.

THE WORKSHEETS

The Grocery List

For easy Lymphomania Weekend prep, print this list and take it with you when you go to your local health food and grocery stores. Remember that not all of the items are essential. Purchase only the foods, nutrients, herbs, and items for the spa treatments you've selected.

Foods

Here are the lymph-boosting foods you'll need. Also, make sure your pantry is stocked with the essential items you learned about in Chapter 2 for any recipes you select.

— cranberries (fresh or frozen)
— cranberry juice (unsweetened)
— flax seeds or flax seed oil
— leafy greens
— nuts and seeds
— sprouts

Nutritional Supplements

— multivitamin and mineral (essential)
— vitamin C (essential)
— protease (optional)

Herbs Selected

Choose one to three of the following herbs:

— astragalus

— cleavers

— echinacea

— wild indigo root

Exercise Equipment

— rebounder

Optional Items If You Selected the Lymph-Boosting Massage Treatment

If you are using the Lymphomania Massage Oil, obtain the following pure essential oils: geranium, juniper, and black pepper. This is optional.

The Lymphomania Weekend Detox Journal

You may wish to print off a copy of the journal page to make it easier to complete.

Energy: Rate your energy (from 0 to 10, with 0 meaning complete exhaustion, and 10 meaning abundant energy). Before the detox _____After the detox _____

Pain: Rate your pain levels (from 0 to 10, with 0 meaning none, and 10 meaning unbearable, constant pain). Before the detox _____ After the detox _____

Mood: Rate your mood (from 0 to 10, with 0 meaning extremely moody, depressed, angry, or irritable, and 10 meaning extremely happy). Before the detox _____ After the detox _____

Weight: Before the detox _____ After the detox _____

Checklist of Lymph-Boosting Foods Consumed

Try to eat at least five a day. Check the ones you ate each day.

	Day 1	Day 2	Day 3
cranberries/cranberry juice	_____	_____	_____
leafy greens	_____	_____	_____
flax seeds/flax seed oil	_____	_____	_____
raw nuts and seeds	_____	_____	_____
sprouts	_____	_____	_____

Selected Nutrients

Be sure to take the multivitamin and extra vitamin C each day. Protease is optional. Write down any additional nutrients you've opted to take throughout the detox. Remember that you don't need to take all of them. Check off each day you take them.

	Day 1	Day 2	Day 3
vitamin C	_____	_____	_____
multivitamin and mineral	_____	_____	_____
protease (optional)	_____	_____	_____

Selected Herbs

Indicate the one to three herbs you've selected to take throughout the detox. Check off each day you take them. Most herbs need to be taken three times daily.

	Day 1	Day 2	Day 3
echinacea	_____	_____	_____
astragalus	_____	_____	_____
cleavers	_____	_____	_____
wild indigo root	_____	_____	_____

Exercise

Check off each time you rebound. Make sure to do it for twenty minutes every day.

	Day 1	Day 2	Day 3
rebounding	_____	_____	_____

Selected Spa Treatment(s)

Check off each time you complete the lymph-boosting spa treatments. It's not necessary to do both of them, but whichever one(s) you choose, make sure you do it every day.

	Day 1	Day 2	Day 3
lymph-boosting massage	_____	_____	_____
dry skin brushing	_____	_____	_____

Observations and Thoughts

Day 1: _____

_____

_____

_____

Day 2: _____

_____

_____

_____

Day 3: _____

_____

_____

_____

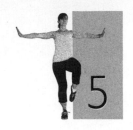

THE KIDNEY FLUSH WEEKEND

BENEFITS OF DETOXIFYING YOUR KIDNEYS
• Fewer urinary tract infections • Less bloating   • Less undereye puffiness   • Less back pain

Your kidneys serve as a first line of defense among detoxification organs. If the kidneys are functioning properly, they reduce the toxic burden on all other organs in your body. The kidneys regulate the body, particularly the water and mineral balance that keeps your cells hydrated. But that's not all. They also excrete toxins in urine and filter and reabsorb substances like minerals in the urine that your body needs. We often link kidney function to waste excretion, but did you know the kidneys also regulate blood pressure through the secretion of hormones?

WHY SHOULD I DETOXIFY MY KIDNEYS?

The consumption of high animal-protein diets like the Standard American Diet (SAD) makes the role of the kidneys even more

GORDON'S BACK PAIN IS DRAMATICALLY REDUCED

Gordon, a middle-aged consultant, came to see me complaining of long-standing back pain. He assumed his back pain was linked to his six-foot-three frame and that few chairs, vehicles, and other elements of life were suited to someone so tall. However, after examining him, I thought there might be other factors at play as well, particularly because he experienced midback pain. In my experience, even if back pain is linked to other factors, kidneys often play a role.

I asked him whether he also experienced frequent urination, a sudden and urgent need to urinate, cloudy urine, or puffiness below his eyes. He indicated that he experienced the former two symptoms on an ongoing basis and the latter two periodically. I shared that I thought his kidneys and urinary tract might need a boost from detoxification. He agreed that he would do the Kidney Flush Weekend and report back after the weekend was over. I outlined the diet, supplements, herbs, exercise, and treatments that I wanted him to follow, and he agreed. I emphasized the importance of drinking more water, which surprised him, considering how much he was already urinating.

Several days later he called me to tell me that he had a significant reduction in the throbbing discomfort, no urgency to urinate but regular urination, and the ability to sit, stand, or drive longer than before and with greater ease and less pain. He also observed that his flexibility was better and that his sleep had improved—both things he never anticipated because he didn't imagine that they were linked to his kidneys. When I asked him how much less pain he felt he indicated that it had improved by about 50 percent. He admitted that such an improvement shocked him and that he planned to maintain many of the changes he had made with the hope that he could eliminate the pain altogether.

I informed him that he could continue any or all of the food and nutritional supplement changes but that he should alternate some of the herbs he was taking to give his body a break from them periodically. He agreed to use bearberry and buchu tea one week and then cleavers and dandelion leaf tea the following week, alternating them each week afterward. I explained that these herbs have diuretic properties, meaning that they

continues

---

continued

eliminate excess water and bloating from the cells and tissues of the body. Although that is beneficial, it was important that he keep taking a multivitamin and mineral supplement to ensure his body obtained sufficient potassium that could otherwise be lost along with the excess water.

He came back to see me six weeks later to share that his back pain was 90 percent improved, with occasional aggravation if he had certain foods like beer or excess sugar. I was impressed that he observed the effects that specific foods had on him, particularly because they usually show up the day after eating them. He explained that having less back pain was motivation enough to keep up many of his newly found healthy habits.

---

important than usual. Unfortunately, these diets make the kidneys work harder as our body tries to metabolize and eliminate these high-protein foods. The kidneys process protein to separate out amino acids for use by the body and to eliminate waste that accumulates from the metabolism of the protein. This includes urea and ammonia, both of which can reach toxic levels if the kidneys can't handle the protein load. This is a problem with many high-protein diets: you will lose weight at first but begin to suffer symptoms of kidney distress. Over time the weight loss will seem unimportant in contrast to the damage that may have occurred to these important detoxification organs.

SIGNS OF STRESSED-OUT KIDNEYS

It is a low-risk gamble to say most people have stressed-out kidneys. Lifestyle stress, exercise, cardiovascular disease, genetic weaknesses, infections, kidney stones, and nutrition levels affect the health of these organs. As I mentioned above, most of us eat too much protein (specifically meat) and drink too little water. Kidneys require water like flowers require water. Dehydration is the most common stress our kidneys face. Without sufficient water, the kidneys won't perform their metabolizing, cleansing, and eliminating functions properly. This is no different from the rest of your body's organs and cells. Without enough clean water, they will become dehydrated and less capable of keeping you healthy.

Salt can be another kidney stressor. Although some sodium is necessary for proper kidney function, too much can be detrimental. Reducing salt intake and increasing the number of potassium-rich foods you eat will help your kidneys do their job. Although not all salt is bad, most salt that people eat is unbalanced in minerals and is essentially a "dead" food. Natural salt should contain sodium along with other minerals like potassium, but during the processing of salt other minerals are removed. And shockingly, sometimes even sugar is added (but that's a story for another day). Choose natural salt like unrefined sea salt, which has a gray color. The color reflects the many minerals present other than just sodium. There are other forms of "natural" salt, but I no longer recommend them. Many forms of crystal salt, for example, can contain lead.

Once you've switched to a more natural form of salt you should still eat salt in moderation. And, if you have high blood pressure, you definitely need to cut back, contrary to what many nutritionists and doctors are advising people these days. The kidneys are intimately involved in controlling blood pressure, and high blood pressure means excessive amounts of sodium and/or insufficient potassium. If you have high blood pressure, you'll also want to eat more potassium-rich foods like green vegetables. Almost all vegetables and fruits are sources of potassium, so eating a plant-based diet like the Kidney Flush Weekend should help. However, high blood pressure may be a sign you'll need to maintain the dietary suggestions for a longer period of time. High blood pressure is not the only sign that you would benefit from a kidney detox.

Signs You Would Benefit from a Kidney Detox

Considering their function, it is not surprising that stressed-out kidneys produce symptoms related to the urinary tract and urination. Bloody, cloudy, or dark-colored urination can all be linked to poor kidney function, as are difficult, frequent or painful urination. Kidney problems are frequently identified with back pain, bloating (including swollen fingers, ankles, and legs), puffiness around the eyes, and chills, fevers, or nausea. Kidney stones are clearly a sign of kidney distress, as is high blood pressure, and serious kidney problems have been linked to both kidney and bladder cancer. Here are some of the symptoms and conditions that are linked to reduced kidney function or a stressed-out urinary tract.

- back pain
- blood in your urine
- cloudy urine
- congestive heart failure
- dark-colored urine
- difficult, frequent, or painful urination
- edema or bloating
- frequent chills, fevers, or nausea
- high blood pressure
- kidney or bladder cancer
- kidney stones
- puffiness around the eyes
- swollen fingers, ankles, legs, and so forth
- urinary tract infections (UTIs)

Although there are many symptoms linked to overburdened kidneys and urinary tract, the flip side of this is that when you strengthen these organs and organ system you will likely see improvements in many conditions.

If you've had serious health issues, you may need longer than the weekend, particularly if you are experiencing an active or ongoing urinary tract infection. Additionally, you may also benefit from following the Colon Cleanse Weekend, as you'll want to ensure rapid elimination of any toxins the Kidney Flush Weekend stirs up.

THE DIET

Although I have touched on general nutrition tips that help or hinder kidney health, there are key foods that your kidneys will love as well as foods that will sabotage these important detoxification organs. In this part of the Kidney Flush Weekend we'll explore the foods to avoid and the best kidney-boosting foods to include in your diet.

Love Your Kidneys Essentials

In addition to the recommendations outlined in Chapter 2, follow these essential guidelines on the Kidney Flush Weekend. Some of the recommendations may overlap, but they are repeated when necessary here in the context of kidney cleansing.

1. **Start every morning with a large glass of water with the fresh juice of one lemon.** Sorry, Realemon or other bottled lemon juice won't do; it must be the real deal. If you can't bear the taste of the lemon water, add a few drops of pure stevia to sweeten it—it will taste like lemonade.

2. **Drink three glasses of cranberry juice or cranberry water daily.** Cranberries and cranberry juice in sufficient quantities can eliminate harmful bacteria in the urinary tract. Their phytonutrients cause bacteria to lose the ability to cling to the walls of the bladder and urinary tract, forcing them out of the body through urine. Research shows that drinking fifteen ounces of pure cranberry juice daily kills about 80 percent of bacterial growth in the urinary tract.[1] If you're just boosting the kidneys and urinary tract health with this cleanse, you won't need to keep up the cranberry juice after the three days; however, if you currently have a urinary tract infection or are prone to recurring infections, then you'll need to keep drinking cranberry juice for at least a month. Use only unsweetened cranberry juice, not cranberry cocktail, which is full of sugar. Alternatively, blend a cup of fresh or frozen cranberries with two cups of water.

3. **Avoid processed, packaged, and prepared foods.** Food additives, colors, artificial sweeteners, preservatives, harmful fats, and artificial ingredients require processing by your kidneys, increasing its workload. Eating them during this weekend will simply negate your best efforts. Eliminating these from your diet gives your kidneys and urinary tract a well-deserved break.

4. **Take a high-quality multivitamin and mineral supplement.** The kidneys and urinary tract require many nutrients to detoxify properly. Even a single nutrient deficiency can be harmful and cause a malfunction in detoxification.

5. **Avoid eating large meals.** Instead, eat small meals made up of plenty of easy-to-digest foods. Your kidneys work tremendously hard to aid digestion. Eating smaller meals frees up energy from digestion for the kidneys to detoxify your body.

6. **Eat lots of vegetables.** We all know we're supposed to eat lots of vegetables, but now is the time to actually do it. Considering it is only for three days, this shouldn't be a problem for anyone. Most of my clients report back that they discover new vegetables and ways of preparing them during the weekend detox that they carry forward throughout their life. Throughout the weekend you can eat vegetables steamed, sautéed, stir-fried, roasted, baked, or raw. Stay clear of fried vegetables.

7. **Eat fish or seaweed daily.** Fish and seaweed are good sources of an important nutrient called docosahexanoic acid (DHA) that helps quell inflammation in the kidneys and urinary tract as well as elsewhere in the body. You'll learn more about this essential fat momentarily, but for now keep in mind that you should eat fish or seaweed daily while doing the Kidney Flush Weekend. For fish, opt for a piece about the size of a deck of cards. For seaweed, aim for a tablespoon if you're using ground or sliced seaweed. If you're choosing nori sheets, one or two sheets daily is perfect. You can also use hijiki, which typically comes in thin, spaghetti-like strands or kelp, both of which can be rehydrated by soaking in water. Either hijiki or kelp is a great addition to soup. There are many types of seaweed available in health food stores. There are even kelp noodles,

which are naturally gluten-free and a delicious, mineral-rich low-carb alternative to high-carb pastas. Kelp noodles are found in the refrigerator section of most health food stores, whereas other types of seaweed are dried and packaged.

8. **Eliminate sugar.** Sugars of any kind, including fruit sugars and so-called natural sweeteners, feed any bacteria or other microbes lingering in your urinary tract and are best avoided this weekend. Eating them during this weekend will simply negate your best cleansing efforts. It's best to avoid fruit other than cranberries this weekend too, especially if you have or are prone to urinary tract infections.

9. **Eat whole, raw, unsalted nuts and seeds.** Nuts and seeds are excellent sources of protein. Without sufficient protein, various processes that comprise liver detoxification can break down or become impaired. Some of your best options include walnuts, almonds, Brazil nuts, pumpkin seeds, sunflower seeds, or sesame seeds. The key is choosing raw and unsalted nuts and seeds. Ideally, they are found in the refrigerator section of your health food store.

10. **Avoid eating heavy, fatty foods.** Heavy, fatty foods bog down all of the digestive and detoxification processes, so they are best avoided this weekend. Avoid margarine, shortening, or commercial oils as well as any foods made with them.

11. **Avoid eating for at least three hours before bedtime.** Your body needs adequate time during the night to perform its many functions, unimpeded by other bodily processes like digestion. This frees up energy to ensure adequate nutrient absorption for the kidneys and to aid the kidneys in performing their detoxification processes.

12. **Drink at least one-half quart or one-half liter (almost the same amount) for every fifty pounds of weight you're carrying, up to about three quarts or liters.** I know this seems like a lot (because it is!), and you may feel like you're spending your weekend in the bathroom, but water is needed to flush toxins from the body. Without sufficient water, toxins can become absorbed

back into the bloodstream, creating a vicious cycle of the kidneys sloughing off toxins, only to have them be reabsorbed into the blood. And try not to drink immediately before or after meals. I know this may be a challenge with all the water you need to drink, but just do your best. Freshly made vegetable and fruit juices count toward your total amount of water. Vegetable juices are preferable to water, as they contain water along with plentiful amounts of vitamins, minerals, phytonutrients, and enzymes. Freshly made fruit juices also contain these beneficial substances but tend to be high in sugars, so they are best consumed in minimal amounts. Canned or bottled vegetable juices are best avoided due to the processing and high amounts of sodium they typically contain. And, of course, cranberry juice or cranberry water count toward your total water intake.

13. **Avoid all carbonated water or soda during the Kidney Flush Weekend.** The high amounts of sugar, artificial sweeteners, or phosphoric acid can be hard on the kidneys. Even so-called health beverages like carbonated water are high in the latter substance. This shouldn't be difficult because the cleanse is only three days, and you'll be drinking a lot of water, cranberry juice, and possibly some vegetable juices.

Dr. Michelle's Top Five Kidney-Boosting Foods

You learned about some of the best kidney-boosting foods earlier in this chapter, but here is more information to help you understand the importance of eating these kidney superfoods.

Cranberries and cranberry juice—Cranberries are excellent for your kidneys. I'm not referring to the processed, sugar-sweetened, artificially flavored version you find in most grocery stores; I'm talking about real cranberries—fresh or frozen—as well as real juice without additives. Although you can use dried cranberry and cranberry supplements, the real deal will give you the substances you need to cleanse your kidneys and urinary tract. These little berries are actually an evergreen shrub, although they are frequently grown in water. In addition to high levels of proanthocyanidins that help prevent damaging bacteria from attaching themselves to the lining of the urinary tract, cranberries contain arbutin, which helps draw excess fluid from tissues. This fluid is eliminated through the kidneys.[2] As an added bonus, cranberries and cranberry juice help break down fatty deposits that can accumulate in the lymphatic system and form cellulite. Learn more about this topic in Chapter 4, "The Lymphomania Weekend."

Fish and seaweed—Fatty fish like wild salmon, anchovies, and sardines contain a kidney-protective fat called docosahexanoic acid (DHA). Tuna, mackerel, and swordfish also contain DHA, but I don't recommend them because they are frequently found to be high in toxins like the heavy metal mercury. Research shows that DHA helps protects the kidneys against toxins and cancer.[3] The same study also found that DHA helps to heal stress and injury to the kidneys, particularly when caused by certain toxins. Eat wild salmon daily on the Kidney Flush Weekend. If you don't like fish, supplement with a DHA (in conjunction with EPA) capsule of 1000mg daily. If you're vegetarian or vegan, you can obtain DHA from seaweed or algae, which should be eaten daily or supplemented daily during the Kidney Flush Weekend. Many vegetarians incorrectly think that flax seeds or walnuts will provide DHA; however, these foods contain essential fatty acids but not DHA.

Green tea—If you haven't started drinking green tea yet, now is the time. It contains potent antioxidants known as epigallocatechin gallate, or EGCG for short. You don't need to be able to pronounce it to reap the benefits of this powerful nutrient, poised to be one of the greatest nutritional discoveries of the decade. EGCG has been shown in multiple studies to protect the kidneys and urinary tract from harmful toxins.[4] It also protects against inflammation some toxins cause.[5] Ideally, drink three cups of green tea daily during your Kidney Flush Weekend. If you don't like the taste of green tea, try my Green Tea Lemonade recipe at the back of the book—I developed the recipe because I really didn't like the taste of green tea. Other green tea haters have told me they love this drink. To enhance green tea's effectiveness, supplement with alpha lipoic acid (see below). The combination has been shown in research to be even more potent.[6]

Turmeric—Not only do taste buds love curries, but kidneys do too. Exciting research in the *Journal of Agricultural Food Chemistry* found that the active ingredient in turmeric—a common curry ingredient—curcumin, is effective at reducing inflammation and damage toxins cause to the kidneys. The scientists involved in the study noted that curcumin had a significant effect on kidney function.[7] Enjoy turmeric in curries, soups, stews, or on its own in some water. For the latter, add one teaspoon of powdered turmeric to a cup of water. Drink—through a straw if possible, as turmeric can stain your teeth. Its kidney-boosting properties are worth it, though, as it helps prevent toxins from damaging the kidneys. For more ideas check out the recipes in Chapter 10 to discover many delicious foods containing turmeric.

THE SUPPLEMENTS

In this section you'll discover the best nutrients and herbs that assist the kidneys with detoxification and healing. You don't need to take all of them—just two or three is great. Reading the following section may give you some insight into which ones might be best for you. Follow the dosage recommendations mentioned later in this section to maximize the kidney-cleansing benefits of your chosen nutrients.

Critical Nutrients for Kidney Cleansing

There are many essential nutrients needed to ensure healthy kidneys. Even a single deficiency can impair proper cleansing or make the urinary tract vulnerable to infection and may result in seemingly unrelated but uncomfortable symptoms.

Most people simply need a high-quality multiple vitamin and mineral with some added vitamin C and probiotics. If you have many of the conditions in the list above, you may need a bit more kidney support. Keep reading to learn whether you might benefit from supplementing with additional nutrients. But don't worry: the last thing I want is for you to be popping handfuls of supplements; choose the ones that make the most sense for you.

Boost Your Kidneys with Probiotics

Contrary to what most people believe, probiotics, or healthy bacteria, are not just for improving bowel function and digestion; they are also beneficial to restoring healthy function to the kidneys and urinary tract. New research in the *Archives of Internal Medicine* shows that two probiotics are almost as effective as antibiotics at eliminating urinary tract infections from the body.[8] But not just any probiotics will do; the specific strains of probiotics known as *Lactobacillus rhamnosus* and *Lactobacillus reuteri*, taken twice daily on an empty stomach for a year, caused a 51.4 percent drop in harmful E. coli bacteria linked to urinary tract infections. And unlike the antibiotics, there are no harmful side effects of taking the probiotics. And because antibiotic drugs are quite simplistic in chemical structure when compared with probiotics, it's no surprise that harmful bacteria are able to "figure them out" and become resistant in a surprisingly short time. Harmful bacteria do not become resistant to probiotics.

Choose a probiotic supplement, either in powder or capsule form, that contains *Lactobacilli rhamnosus* and *reuteri*. Take two capsules or one-half teaspoon on an empty stomach, about twenty minutes before eating. First thing in the morning is ideal. I take them and then go have my shower and get ready for the day. Many people ask me whether they can just eat yogurt. Although yogurt is beneficial, it rarely provides the strains of bacteria needed for kidney rejuvenation.

Beat Infection with Vitamin C

When it comes to the kidneys and urinary tract, not only does vitamin C give them a boost, but it also inhibits the growth of harmful bacteria like E. coli and others to prevent infections. Take 1000mg five times a day, in divided doses, to boost your kidneys and to help kill any infections in your urinary tract. Because ascorbic acid can be irritating to the bladder, choose calcium ascorbate instead. If you are suffering from a urinary tract infection or are prone to recurring ones, you may need higher doses of vitamin C to sufficiently kill any lingering bacteria—sometimes as much as 10,000 or 15,000mg daily are needed. Don't worry: there are no ill effects of taking such high doses of vitamin C, particularly when it is taken in doses of 1000 to 2000mg at a time. That's because vitamin C is water soluble, meaning that any excess is eliminated in your urine. The higher concentration of vitamin C in your urine goes to work killing harmful bacteria in the urinary tract. If you experience loose bowel movements, that means you've just surpassed the dose that's ideal for you and should back down by about 1000mg.

Boost Your Kidneys with Magnesium

Responsible for hundreds of biochemical processes in your body, including various ones involved in healthy kidney and urinary tract function, magnesium is essential during the Kidney Flush Weekend (and even after it is over). A deficiency of magnesium has been linked to kidney stones. According to Carolyn Dean, MD, ND, and author of *The Miracle of Magnesium*, approximately 80 percent of the North American population are deficient in magnesium.[9] I recommend magnesium glycinate. About 800mg daily is ideal during the Kidney Flush Weekend.

Heal Your Kidneys with Alpha Lipoic Acid

One of the most potent healing nutrients is also one of the most underrated. Alpha lipoic acid (or ALA, or sometimes just called lipoic acid) not only functions as a superpowerful antioxidant that is much stronger than most antioxidants; it also recycles other antioxidants to keep them protecting your body against free radical damage much longer than they otherwise could. In other words, it keeps antioxidants like vitamins A, C, and E working long after they would have retired. And exciting new research shows that it is especially good at preventing and healing inflammation and damage to the kidneys, particularly when taken along with green tea or its active ingredient, EGCG.[10] A typical dose for alpha lipoic acid is 100mg, and green tea extract is 300mg.

More Kidney-Boosting Nutritional Supplements

I recommend a high-quality multivitamin and mineral supplement that contains vitamins A, C, and E as well as potassium and zinc. Vitamin A helps to heal the urinary tract lining, and vitamin C acidifies urine to prevent stones from forming. Vitamin E is an antioxidant that protects all your cells, including your kidney cells, from free radical damage. Potassium acts as a kidney stimulant, and zinc slows down crystallization to decrease the likelihood of kidney stone formation.

Herbal Kidney Boosters

As always, Mother Nature provides great herbal remedies for kidney health and welfare. These herbs can be found in the wild, in your backyard garden, and even in your lawn. However, if you're not an experienced wild-crafter who can recognize the plants, it is best to purchase the herbs you'll be using from a reputable health food store or herbal supplier. Some of the best herbal kidney and urinary tract cleansers include bearberry, buchu, cleavers, and dandelion.

Bearberry (Arctostaphylos uva ursi)

An effective kidney and urinary tract cleanser, this herb can also reduce inflammation if it is present in these areas. In addition to helping with infections and kidney stones or gravel, bearberry can also combat vaginal infections and vaginitis. Use only the amount directed below, as larger doses should be avoided because they can cause nausea and vomiting; however, a teaspoon of dried bearberry leaves steeped in a cup of boiling water for twenty minutes will do the trick. You should try to drink a cup of bearberry tea three times a day.

Buchu (Agathosma betulina)

Buchu also makes a great kidney tea. By following the same recipe and dosage for bearberry above, your buchu tea will help increase urinary flow, which in turn will help eliminate toxins from the body. Unlike many other herbs that have healing properties on different parts of the body, buchu has its best results on the kidneys and urinary tract. It is effective against cystitis, prostatitis, burning or painful urination, and urethritis.

Cleavers (Galium aparine)

Cleavers, which also goes by the name "goosegrass" or "grip grass," helps the kidney flush out toxins and waste fluids and reduces the toxic load within the tissues. Although individuals with diabetes or diabetic tendencies should avoid cleavers, others can enjoy it in tea or tincture forms. Two or three teaspoons of the dried herb in boiling water make one cup of tea. Three cups a day will get your kidneys feeling great. If you find cleavers in a tincture form at your health store, follow the instructions up to one teaspoon three times a day.

Dandelion (Taraxacum officinale)

These "weeds" are not only one of the best detoxification and healing herbs; they are also nutrient-packed powerhouses containing protein, vitamins A and C, iron, and minerals. The entire plant is edible and medicinal, although you should not eat dandelions if the areas in which they grow have been sprayed with weed killers and other pesticides. If you live in an area where you know the soil is clean and chemicals are not used, you may have a treasure trove of kidney-cleansing dandelions at your disposal.

Dandelion leaves are the best part of the plant for kidney health. The young leaves of the plant are tender and make excellent

additions to salads. The root is also effective, but it is more beneficial for liver detoxification and is discussed for that purpose in the
Love Your Liver Weekend chapter. One teaspoon of dried leaves
per cup of hot water makes an excellent infusion. Like the teas
above, drink one cup three times a day. Dandelion is a natural diuretic; however, it contains potassium and calcium to prevent mineral depletion that is so common with pharmaceutical diuretics.

If you have gallstones or obstructed bile ducts, consult with a
holistic physician before adding dandelion to your diet.

THE EXERCISE

Leg Sweep and Swing

The Leg Sweep and Swing exercise helps get energy in the kidneys, bladder, and urinary system flowing to flush out toxins, eliminate infection, and to boost their health. This is a simple exercise
that is based on a system of yoga called Dahn Yoga, as outlined in
the excellent book *Meridian Exercise for Self-Healing* by Ilchi Lee.[11]
Perform this exercise once or twice daily during the Kidney Flush
Weekend.

To perform the exercise, stand with your feet wide apart. They
should be wider apart than your shoulder width. Place your hands
behind your back at waist level as shown in Figure 5.1. Take a deep
breath in. Bend your body at the hips while dragging your hands
down the backs of your legs until you can grasp your ankles. Then
gently pull your upper body toward your ankles until your head is
between your feet. Don't worry if you can't quite reach that far.
Don't strain, but do go a bit farther than is comfortable. Practice
makes perfect. Hold this posture for about ten seconds (or longer if
you can). Then exhale and return to the starting position. Repeat
until you've completed this part of the exercise three times.

Now, stand normally with your hands on your waist. Lift your
right leg, and flex your foot while keeping your knees straight
but soft. Swing your leg forward and backward behind your back
twenty times on each leg. See Figures 5.3 and 5.4.

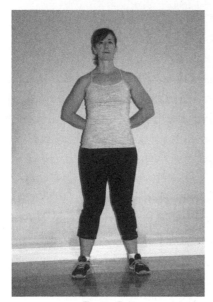

Figure 5.1

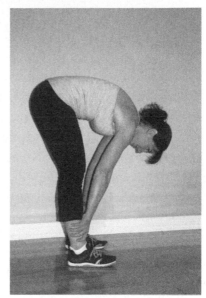

Figure 5.2

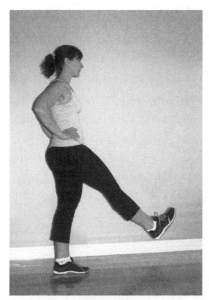

Figure 5.3

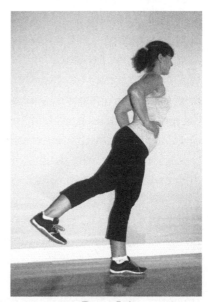

Figure 5.4

THE SPA TREATMENTS

Healthy Kidney Meditation

The kidneys not only play a significant role in balancing minerals (sodium and potassium), blood pressure, and even our body's pH level; they are also connected to the adrenal glands, which are two triangular-shaped glands that sit atop the kidneys and are often called the stress glands because they regulate our reaction to stress but can also become worn down with excessive stress.

Some natural health experts believe that kidney issues can be the result of feeling disempowered and not feeling in control of your life or from not having a say in your life as you were growing up. It can also be linked with setting boundaries, saying "no" to people or obligations in life. Sometimes it is essential to say "no" to do what is best for your health and wellness.

You can heal the kidneys through meditation, making them impermeable to negative influences. Here's a simple color meditation to boost your kidneys.

Sit or lie down in a comfortable position, making sure your back is straight. Take a few moments to get settled, and begin by observing your breath. Is it shallow or deep? Is it strong or weak? Don't try to force your breathing, but visualize your breath moving into your solar plexus in your stomach, just under your ribs. What do you feel in this area? Is it tight or relaxed? Do you feel nervousness, anxiety, or other emotions held in your body?

Gradually breathe deeper, but don't force it. Let your breathing deepen slowly and naturally. Visualize life-giving oxygen entering your diaphragm just below your ribs. See toxins leaving this area and your body, floating out into the Universe where they can be recycled. In their place see brilliant yellow light entering your body through your solar plexus region just below your ribs. When it feels right, begin to visualize the yellow light swirling clockwise. Imagine this yellow swirling energy is cleansing your body of all anger, jealousy, stress, and any other emotion that may be holding you back. Now they are replaced by healing and positive feelings of strength, tranquility, peace, and harmony.

Continue doing this meditation for as long as you would like. When it feels right, slowly open your eyes and sit or stand up, remembering to continue breathing deeply as you go about your day. You can perform this meditation repeatedly during the Kidney Flush Weekend or any time you feel like you need a boost of energy or a cleansing of negative emotions. Perform the Healthy Kidney Meditation at least once daily during the Kidney Flush Weekend. You can do this meditation as much as you'd like even after the detox.

Acupressure for Kidney Detox and Healing

As you learned in Chapter 2, there are points along energy pathways that supply the organs in the body with the energy they need to function properly. The points at which these pathways surface are called acupressure points, or acupoints. To supercharge your kidney and urinary tract cleansing efforts, use the acupressure points indicated below.

Apply firm pressure to the points. Hold each one for a minute or two. You can work on both sides simultaneously or do one side at a time, whichever suits you best. For example, Kidney 1 (K1) is located in a slight depression beneath the balls of both feet (as seen in Figure 5.5 below). You can apply pressure to this point on both feet at the same time or hold one at a time if that is easier for you.

I've listed four sets of two points. Don't worry if you're not sure whether you're finding the right points—just do your best. If you find points that feel a bit tender, you've probably found the points that are needed. If you are pregnant, avoid using the point Stomach 36 (St36) and consult with an acupuncturist before proceeding with acupressure.

You'll see that the points are grouped in sets of two. Feel free to hold both points at once. For example, you can hold both Liver 1 and Kidney 1 at the same time.

Use the following points:

Liver 1 (Liv1) is located on the edge of the big toe near the bottom corner of the toenail, on the edge near the second toe.

Kidney 1 (K1) is located on the base of the ball of the foot. This point is found in a slight depression.

Then:

Spleen 3 (Sp3) is located on the inside of the foot, at the base of the protrusion behind the big toe.

Kidney 5 (K5) is located just behind the ankle bone, on the inside of the foot.

Then:

Gallbladder 41 (GB41) is located on the top of the foot toward the outside edge, about an inch and a half above the fourth toe (the toe nearest the little toe).

Urinary Bladder 65 (UB65) is located on the outside edge of the foot, about an inch below the base of the little toe.

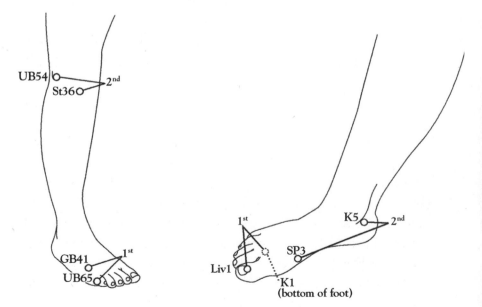

Figure 5.5

Then:

Stomach 36 (St36) is located in the space where the two lower leg bones meet just below and to the outer edge of the kneecap.

Urinary Bladder 54 (UB54) is located toward the outside edge of the base of the knee.

You may be wondering, *Why would I use liver, gallbladder, spleen, and stomach points when I'm trying to boost my urinary tract and kidneys?* There are multiple reasons for this.

1. The points often have multiple functions beyond what is evident by the name of the points.
2. The points often intersect a related channel of energy flow and can thereby supply energy to the kidneys and urinary tract.
3. Boosting the strength of another organ or organ system can add support to the kidneys. For example, the liver supports detoxification and must pick up the slack when the kidneys are overwhelmed. Boosting this important organ gives the kidneys added support in dealing with toxins.

THE WEEKEND

You are now quite familiar with the kidneys and urinary tract, the foods that strengthen it, and the nutrients, herbs, exercises, and spa treatments that give it a boost. Here's where we'll put the whole program together to make it easier for you.

I've outlined a step-by-step approach to the Kidney Flush Weekend detox below. Of course, you can substitute other foods. The schedule and meal plan are just guidelines, so feel free to adjust them to suit your preferences. Just be sure you've included the foods, herbs, and essential dietary guidelines into your weekend. If it is easier for you to drink an herbal tea, then feel free to use the Kidney Herbal Tea recipe in the Recipes section. If you drink this tea three times daily, you'll have met the herbal requirements and won't need to take additional herbs.

Here's what your three-day Kidney Flush Weekend will look like:

Days one to three:

Upon rising—Cranberry Pear Juice (page 242), Cranberry Green Tea Lemonade (page 243), or one cup of fresh or frozen cranberries blended with one cup of water. Add a few drops of liquid stevia if you prefer a sweeter-tasting beverage. Wait twenty minutes before eating.

Exercise—leg sweep and swing

Breakfast—Be sure to include some of the kidney-boosting foods mentioned above. Some good options include Kidney Herbal Tea (page 246), Veggie Scramble (page 262), a soft-boiled egg with Lemon-Garlic Greens (page 252), or cooked brown rice with almond milk.

Multivitamin

Optional nutrients

Herb (first dose of selected herbs)

Midmorning—Large glass of water (with lemon if desired), a cup of Kidney Herbal Tea (page 246), or Super-Detoxifying Green Tea Lemonade (page 243)

Snack, such as an apple with almond butter, raw unsalted walnuts, or celery sticks with almond butter or Herbes de Provence Cashew Cheese (page 250)

Acupressure for kidney detox and healing

Lunch—Weekend Wonder Detox Signature Salad (page 258) or other large detoxifying salad topped with seaweed (page 254)

Cranberry Pear Juice (page 242) or Honey-Turmeric Tea (page 247)

Vitamin C

Optional nutrients

Herb (second dose of selected herbs)

Midafternoon—Large glass of water (with lemon if desired), a cup of Kidney Herbal Tea (page 246), or Honey-Turmeric Tea (page 247)

Snack, such as a grapefruit, apple, raw unsalted walnuts, or celery sticks with almond butter

Dinner—Lentil Bowl with a teaspoon of turmeric added (page 263) with Lemon-Garlic Greens (page 252) or Curried Garbanzo Bean and Squash Stew (page 265)

Fresh cup of Kidney Herbal Tea (page 246) or Carrot Celery Juice (page 240)

Herb (third dose of selected herb)

After dinner—Cantaloupe Ice (page 241) or two Pumpkin Spice Drop Cookies (page 267)

Healthy kidney meditation

Before bed—Take some quiet time to turn off the television. Find a quiet place to sit, close your eyes, and take some deep breaths.

Write in the Kidney Flush Weekend Detox Journal (at the end of this chapter)

CONCLUDING THE KIDNEY FLUSH WEEKEND

You just gave your kidneys and urinary tract a wonderful boost, which in turn can help the health of your whole body. Completing the Kidney Flush Weekend is something you should feel proud of.

I encourage you to keep incorporating foods, nutrients, herbs, exercises, or spa treatments into your day-to-day life after the detox is over. Your kidneys help detoxify your whole body, so it is important to continue nurturing them throughout life.

You may wish to do the Kidney Flush Weekend every weekend for a month or one weekend out of every month. The choice is yours. You know your lifestyle and schedule best. Choose the option that works best for you.

If you continue to follow the Kidney Flush Weekend for longer periods, every three weeks just take one week off from any herbs you're using.

And be sure to try some of the other health-building weekend detoxes I've included throughout *Weekend Wonder Detox*. If you're still feeling tired and worn out, try the Colon Cleanse Weekend next.

THE WORKSHEETS

The Grocery List

For easy Kidney Flush weekend prep, print this list and take it with you when you go to your local health food and grocery stores. Remember that not all of the items are essential. Purchase only the foods, nutrients, herbs, and items for the spa treatments you've selected.

Foods

Here are the kidney-boosting foods you'll need. Also, make sure your pantry is stocked with the essential items you learned about in Chapter 2 for any recipes you select.

— cranberries (fresh or frozen)

— cranberry juice (unsweetened)

— fish (wild salmon, anchovies, or sardines)

— seaweed/sea vegetables

— green tea (if you prefer my green tea lemonade, then you'll also need liquid stevia and lemons)

— turmeric

Nutritional Supplements

— multivitamin and mineral (essential)

— probiotics (be sure it contains *Lactobacillus rhamnosus* and *Lactobacillus reuteri*) (essential)

— vitamin C (essential)

— magnesium (optional)

— alpha lipoic acid (ALA—optional)

Herbs Selected

Choose one to three of the following herbs:

— bearberry

— buchu

— cleavers

— dandelion leaves

The Kidney Flush Weekend Detox Journal

You may wish to print off a copy of the journal page to make it easier to complete.

Energy: Rate your energy (from 0 to 10, with 0 meaning complete exhaustion, and 10 meaning abundant energy). Before the detox _____ After the detox _____

Pain: Rate your pain levels (from 0 to 10, with 0 meaning none, and 10 meaning unbearable, constant pain). Before the detox _____ After the detox _____

Mood: Rate your mood (from 0 to 10, with 0 meaning extremely moody, depressed, angry, or irritable, and 10 meaning extremely happy). Before the detox _____ After the detox _____

Weight: Before the detox _____ After the detox _____

Checklist of Kidney-Boosting Foods Consumed

Try to eat at least five a day. Check the ones you ate each day.

	Day 1	Day 2	Day 3
cranberries (fresh or frozen)	_____	_____	_____
cranberry juice (unsweetened)	_____	_____	_____
fish (wild salmon, sardines, anchovies)	_____	_____	_____
seaweed/sea vegetables	_____	_____	_____
green tea	_____	_____	_____
turmeric	_____	_____	_____

Selected Nutrients

Be sure to take the multivitamin, probiotics, and vitamin C each day. Write down any additional nutrients you've opted to take throughout the detox. Remember that you don't need to take all of them. Check off each day you take them.

	Day 1	Day 2	Day 3
multivitamin and mineral	_____	_____	_____
probiotics	_____	_____	_____
vitamin C	_____	_____	_____
magnesium (optional)	_____	_____	_____
green tea	_____	_____	_____
alpha lipoic acid (optional)	_____	_____	_____

Selected Herbs

Indicate the one to three herbs you've selected to take throughout the detox. Check off each day you take them. Most herbs need to be taken three times daily.

	Day 1	Day 2	Day 3
bearberry	_____	_____	_____
buchu	_____	_____	_____
cleavers	_____	_____	_____
dandelion (leaves)	_____	_____	_____

Exercise

Check off each time you complete the leg sweep and swing. Make sure to do it every day.

	Day 1	Day 2	Day 3
Leg sweep and swing	_____	_____	_____

Selected Spa Treatment(s)

Check off each time you complete the kidney-boosting spa treatments. It's not necessary to do both of them, but whichever one(s) you choose, make sure you do it every day.

	Day 1	Day 2	Day 3
healthy kidney meditation	_____	_____	_____
acupressure for kidney detox and healing	_____	_____	_____

Observations and Thoughts

Day 1: _____

_____

_____

_____

Day 2: _____

_____

_____

_____

Day 3: _____

_____

_____

_____

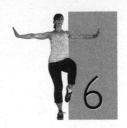

THE COLON CLEANSE WEEKEND

BENEFITS OF DETOXIFYING YOUR INTESTINES	
• Less bloating	• Lighter feeling
• Flatter abdomen	• Less back pain
• Improved bowel regularity	• Improved immune system
• Less abdominal discomfort	• Improved digestion

What happens in Vegas may stay in Vegas, but what happens in your colon shouldn't stay there—for good reason. What happens in your bowels determines the health of every other part of your body. This may seem odd or even a bit disgusting to some people, but it is true. Seemingly unrelated parts of your body can be intimately connected. When it comes to your health it is more accurately reflected as "what happens in your bowels determines the health of your brain, immune system, blood, and every other bodily system." In short, keeping your intestines functioning smoothly will help keep your body strong against toxins, help maintain a strong system, improve your nutritional status, and help keep every part of your body healthy.

BOBBI OVERCOMES BOWEL IMBALANCES

Bobbi was diagnosed with irritable bowel syndrome as a young teenager. Her doctor informed her that she would likely have bowel troubles for the rest of her life and that she may need additional medical intervention "down the road."

Although most people accept a doctor's diagnosis and prognosis as a sort of life sentence, Bobbi refused to accept that. She explained that she couldn't imagine that the same body that healed wounds and bones could just stop working properly when it came to the bowels. This no-nonsense young woman intuitively knew that nature must have the answers. In most health issues the body is trying to get our attention to let us know that we're doing something that is not harmonious with nature.

Bobbi ate a typical North American diet: meat, potatoes, pasta, some vegetables, and desserts. Bobbi, like most people, was not getting enough fiber or high-water foods. She ate more meat, poultry, and eggs than her body needed even though it was still growing and she needed more protein foods than a fully developed adult would need.

Bobbi agreed to eat a plant-based diet for the long weekend and to do the Colon Cleanse Weekend. She believed it held the answers to her bloating, indigestion, cramping, and alternating diarrhea and constipation. She called me the next day, worried that she felt a bit more bloated than usual and that she was having loose bowel movements. I explained that her body was adjusting to a higher water and fiber diet and that this was completely normal, albeit a bit uncomfortable. I asked her to stick with it. After the third day of the Colon Cleanse Weekend Bobbi called to tell me that her bowels already felt "cleaner" and that the bloating had subsided. She wasn't experiencing any cramping or other uncomfortable symptoms she had experienced prior to starting the cleanse. She even felt "lighter."

However, a week later, when she drank milk again, the uncomfortable intestinal symptoms started again. Bobbi clearly had trouble with milk (most people do, but they don't make the link to milk or dairy consumption). She then avoided dairy altogether and again had no signs of an irritable bowel. Her physical improvements made her decide to do the Colon Cleanse Weekend every other month while maintaining many of the dietary suggestions in between. She was proud that she trusted her instincts regarding the healing power of nature.

Once you've experienced the Colon Cleanse Weekend you'll understand why Bobbi was so enthusiastic about the health improvements she experienced. Obviously, for longstanding bowel imbalances you'll need more than a weekend, but the Colon Cleanse Weekend is a great way to eliminate toxins from your intestines before they can become reabsorbed into your blood and circulate throughout your body.

WHY SHOULD I DETOXIFY MY INTESTINES?

There are many reasons why the health of your intestines plays an enormous role in your overall health. You are what you eat, according to the old adage. But I think "you are what you digest, absorb, and assimilate" is an important addition to the saying. After all, what you eat, digest, absorb, and assimilate will become the building blocks of every cell in your body, whether it is your heart, brain, muscles, or any other part of your body. If the digestion process is impaired, your body will lack adequate building blocks to maintain healthy cells. It's that simple. Surprising as it may be, your intestines determine what you digest, absorb, and assimilate, at least in part.

Research is showing that the gastrointestinal tract (GI), which includes the small and large intestines, plays a huge part in your body's immune response. It is one of the main determinants of the levels of inflammation in your body and whether your body will attack healthy tissue. This has far-reaching implications for your health. It plays a role in whether you will maintain a healthy immune system, suffer from frequent cold or flu viruses, or suffer from a serious immune system impairment. A healthy immune system is needed to fight infections, but it also determines whether you will have rheumatoid arthritis, a properly functioning thyroid gland, and even lupus.

Nutrients are absorbed through the lining of the intestines to gain direct access to the blood. That's because nutrients are essential to life. Inadequate amounts of nutrients means a breakdown in some aspect of health. When bowel function slows or is impaired in some way the fecal matter that is lodged in the pockets of the intestinal walls blocks nutrient absorption. Additionally, when fecal matter is lodged in the intestines, the toxic material found in fecal matter actually travels across the intestinal wall in place of nutrients to gain direct access to the blood, where these toxins will travel to various organs like the liver, kidneys, and even the brain. So maintaining clean intestines can significantly stop toxins' ability to damage cells, tissues, or organs in the body. It is, therefore, the first line of defense against toxins.

Intestinal cleansing helps keep you regular. Research shows that constipation or fewer than one bowel movement daily is linked to disease. This is especially true of breast disease and breast cancer. A study in the medical journal the *Lancet* found a link between poor intestinal health and breast disease. Women who had daily bowel movements had fewer incidences of breast disease than those who didn't, and women who had two or fewer bowel movements weekly had four times the likelihood of breast disease.[1] Another study in the *American Journal of Public Health* found an increased incidence of breast cancer among women who had infrequent bowel movements, hard stools, or constipation.[2]

Microbiome in the Balance

Over 100 trillion bacteria of more than four hundred different species reside in your intestines. Actually, there are more microorganisms found in your digestive tract than there are cells in your body. Most of these bacteria reside in the large intestine, which is also known as the colon. We tend to become alarmed at the very thought of bacteria residing in our bodies, but these bacteria are an important part of our health; they help ensure that food is adequately broken down, nutrients are synthesized and absorbed, toxins are not absorbed into the blood, harmful bacteria stay in check, and that the immune system is healthy. These beneficial bacteria are also known as flora, microflora, or probiotics (the opposite of antibiotics).

The two main categories of beneficial bacteria, which are also called "friendly bacteria," include lactobacilli and bifidobacteria. Research is beginning to show that these two types of microflora can lower the levels of toxic compounds that could have detrimental effects on the brain. So it is important to make sure there is a healthy balance of these healthy bacteria so they can keep harmful bacteria in check. We all have some degree of harmful bacteria in our intestines, but it is the ratio of the good to bad bacteria that matters. That's what we refer to as the microbiome, or biome for short. The beneficial bacteria not only help ensure the proper breakdown of food and absorption of nutrients through the intestinal walls (that's where most nutrients are absorbed) and into the blood; they also help manufacture some critical nutrients like vitamin B-12, which your body needs to ensure healthy blood and sufficient energy to perform all of its cellular tasks. Studies show that these beneficial bacteria also lower immune system compounds called cytokines not only in the gut but also throughout the bloodstream. Cytokines are linked to anxiety, symptoms of depression, and cognitive disturbances even in healthy adults. Cytokines also lower levels of an important brain and nerve cell protector.

Healthy bacteria in the bowels can also act as antioxidants in the body. Several studies demonstrate the importance of restoring bowel bacterial balance. Healthy bacterial balance in the intestines has a protective ability against free radical damage, especially against damage to the fatty component of cells. Because the brain is largely fat, protecting the fatty component of cells from free radical damage is important to brain health too. The intestines are so important to your brain health that many health professionals are now calling the intestines the "second brain."

THE DIET

Cleansing your intestines may seem daunting, but it's much easier than you think. It is imperative that you follow the dietary suggestions below as closely as possible. Here are the ten Colon Cleanse Weekend essentials to get the best results from your cleanse.

SIGNS YOU WOULD BENEFIT
FROM AN INTESTINAL CLEANSE

Here are some of the symptoms and conditions that are linked to toxic buildup or bacterial overgrowth in the intestines that may also indicate that you would benefit from the Colon Cleanse Weekend:

Some of the symptoms and disorders that are often linked to an imbalance of microorganisms within the intestines include:[3]

abdominal pain or cramping

acne

allergies

anxiety

any disorder of the
   digestive tract

autoimmune disorders
   (rheumatoid arthritis, lupus,
   Hashimoto's thyroiditis, etc.)

back pain (especially lower to
   midback)

bad breath

bloating

burping

"brain fog"

brittle nails or hair

chronic fatigue syndrome
   (diagnosed by a doctor)

coated tongue

constipation

diarrhea

eczema or psoriasis

fatigue

fibromyalgia

flatulence

food sensitivities

frequent sore throats

heartburn

hemorrhoids

high cholesterol

indigestion

irritable bowel syndrome

liver dysfunction

mood swings

multiple allergic response
   syndrome (MARS)

multiple food allergies

muscle or joint pain

nausea and bloating

premenstrual syndrome (PMS)

prostate disorders

sinus infections

sluggish lymphatic system

sore or bleeding gums

yeast infections or vaginitis

The Colon Cleanse Weekend Essentials

1. **Start every morning with a glass of water and two probiotic supplement capsules or one teaspoon of probiotic powder.** I'll discuss probiotic supplements more momentarily.

2. **Wait at least twenty minutes and then follow up with a cup or two of warm water with the fresh juice of one lemon squeezed into it.** Realemon or other bottled lemon juice won't do—it must be the real deal. If you can't bear the tart taste, you can add a few drops of pure stevia to sweeten it.

3. **Avoid processed, packaged, and prepared foods.** Any food additives, colors, artificial sweeteners, preservatives, or harmful fats need to be broken down by your detoxification organs and then eliminated via the intestines, so avoiding them helps to ensure that they cannot do damage in your intestines or, worse, cannot be absorbed via the lining of the intestines into your blood. These foods tend to inflame and clog the intestines, so there is no place for them in an intestinal cleansing weekend.

4. **Increase the amount of raw foods in your diet.** Raw fruit, vegetables, sprouts, and herbs contain the enzymes needed to digest them, thereby freeing up your body's energy. These foods also tend to be high in water, which is critical to proper elimination in the bowels.

5. **Make sure you are eating at least thirty-five grams of fiber daily.** Fiber literally sweeps your intestines clean. I've included my picks for the Top Colon-Cleansing Foods below along with the amount of fiber in each. Make sure you're eating enough of these powerhouse cleansing foods to reach the thirty-five grams of fiber daily. It's easier than you think.

6. **Avoid gluten for the next few days.** For those people with serious intestinal or autoimmune conditions, you may want to keep going after the Colon Cleanse Weekend is done. You may recall the gluten-free grains that were outlined in Chapter 2.

7. **Drink at least one-half quart or one-half liter (they're almost the same amount) for every fifty pounds of weight you're**

carrying up to about three quarts or liters. I know this seems like a lot (because it is!) and you may feel like you're spending your weekend in the bathroom, but you need water to flush toxins from your body. Without sufficient water, toxins can be absorbed back into the bloodstream, creating a vicious cycle of the sloughed-off toxins getting reabsorbed into the blood. And try not to drink immediately before or after meals. Freshly made vegetable and fruit juices count toward your total amount of water. Vegetable juices are preferable to water because they contain water along with plentiful amounts of vitamins, minerals, phytonutrients, and enzymes. Freshly made fruit juices also contain these beneficial substances but tend to be high in sugars, so they are best consumed in minimal amounts. Yes, you may feel a bit bloated from this much water, but if you're experiencing bloated or swollen tissues, it usually means that you may be dehydrated.

8. **Avoid drinking with meals or drink only enough to take medications or supplements.** Water increases the pH of the stomach, which prematurely neutralizes stomach acid and signals the body to move the food into the intestines, even if it is insufficiently digested. And the intestines cannot do the job of the stomach. That sends undigested or partially digested food to the intestines. When this happens nutrients cannot be absorbed across the intestinal walls into the blood, so we start to experience nutritional deficiencies, no matter how well we eat or how many supplements we take. Drinking a lot of water is essential to the Colon Cleanse Weekend, just not with meals. Wait at least twenty minutes after drinking water to eat and about one hour after meals to drink again.

9. **Snack on healthy snacks between meals.** Some snack ideas include raw, unsalted nuts and seeds or celery sticks with almond butter or hummus. These snacks help increase the amount of fiber you're getting to help you reach the 35 grams goal, which we'll discuss in greater detail momentarily.

10. **Avoid eating for at least three hours before bed.** Take another dose of two probiotic capsules or one teaspoon of probiotic powder with a small glass of water.

Dr. Michelle's Top Colon-Cleansing Foods

There are so many great intestinal cleansing foods that picking only ten or twelve is difficult. Instead, I've selected the best categories of colon-cleansing foods. Try to eat at least one food from each category every day for the three days of the Colon Cleanse Weekend. In other words, choose one legume, one nut (unless you're allergic, of course), one seed, one berry, and so forth. All of the grains listed under the "Grains" category are gluten-free, so you can enjoy them even if you are sensitive to gluten or have celiac disease. The number beside each food indicates the amount of fiber in each, so do your best to eat thirty-five grams of fiber daily too.

Legumes

When it comes to cleansing your intestines, beans really are the "magical fruit" of the old children's adage. Once you see how much fiber they contain you'll understand why. For each, the amount of grams of fiber refers to one cup of cooked beans.

adzuki beans	17
black beans	15
black turtle beans	17
broad beans (fava)	9
French beans	17
garbanzo beans (chickpeas)	12
kidney beans	16
lentils	16
lima beans	14
mung beans	15
navy beans	19
pinto beans	15
white beans (small)	19
yellow beans	18

Nuts

The following lists the number of grams of fiber in a one-ounce serving of nuts. You may also notice that peanuts are not listed. Most peanuts contain aflatoxins (a type of mold) that is inflammatory and harmful to the body, so peanuts are best avoided during your colon cleanse.

almonds	4
Brazil nuts	12
cashews	1
pine nuts	12
pistachios	3
walnuts	2

Seeds

The humble seed is actually one of the healthiest foods you can eat. Seeds tend to have a high amount of protein per unit of weight as well as being a rich source of healthy oils and essential fats. And of course, they are also a good source of fiber. I've listed the serving size needed to obtain the number of grams of fiber listed below:

chia seeds (two tablespoons)	10
flax seeds (two tablespoons)	4
hemp seeds (two tablespoons)	2
pumpkin seeds (one-half cup)	3
sunflower seeds (one-quarter cup)	3
sesame seeds (one-quarter cup)	4

Berries

Berries are some of the best colon cleansers not only because they are high in fiber but also because they are typically eaten raw, so the natural enzymes are left intact. Additionally, they are high in phytonutrients like proanthocyanidins, which protect your body against many different diseases. The amount of fiber is grams per cup of fresh or frozen berries. Sorry, canned berries are not part of the Colon Cleanse Weekend.

blackberries	8
blueberries	4
boysenberries	7
currants (red or white)	5
elderberries	10
gooseberries	6
loganberries	8
raspberries	8
strawberries	3

Grains

Grains tend to be quite high in fiber and make excellent additions to your diet while cleansing your intestines. You should avoid all refined grains like white rice or wheat. Because many people suffer from gluten or gliaden sensitivity, it is best to stick with gluten-free grains on the Colon Cleanse Weekend. The unit of measure refers to cooked grain unless otherwise indicated and is written in parentheses beside the grain, followed by the number of grams of fiber.

amaranth (one cup)	6
brown rice (one cup)	4
buckwheat groats (one cup)	5
millet (one cup)	2
oats (gluten-free, one-half cup)	4
quinoa (one cup)	5
teff (dry, uncooked) (one-quarter cup)	6
wild rice (one cup)	3

Leafy Greens

Leafy greens are rich in many different nutrients, including beta carotene, calcium, magnesium, and the phytonutrient chlorella.

Additionally, they are high in fiber. If you're just not a fan, try them sautéed in olive oil and fresh garlic, then squeeze fresh lemon over them just before eating—you'll be surprised how delicious greens taste prepared in this simple manner. The amount of fiber is measured in grams and per cup of cooked greens.

beet greens	4
collard greens	5
kale	2.6
mustard greens	5
spinach	4
swiss chard	4
turnip greens	5

Squash

Squashes of all kinds are excellent colon cleansers due to their high fiber content. The number beside each type of squash refers to grams of fiber in one cup of cooked squash.

acorn squash	9
butternut squash	6
hubbard squash	7
spaghetti squash	2
summer squash	5
zucchini squash	3

THE SUPPLEMENTS

In this section you'll discover the best nutrients and herbs that assist the intestines with cleansing, healing, and elimination. You don't need to take all of them—just two or three is great. Reading the following section may give you guidance as to which nutrients and herbs are best suited for your needs. To maximize their benefits, follow the dosage recommendations for each.

Critical Nutrients for Intestinal Cleansing

There are many nutrients needed for healthy detoxification of the intestines, repair of the intestinal lining, and bacterial balance of microbes within the intestines. To help avoid nutritional deficiencies, it is important to take a high-quality multiple vitamin and mineral supplement on a daily basis. Be sure it is free of gluten, sweeteners, artificial sweeteners, colors, preservatives, and fillers.

The health of the intestines is also dependent on sufficient gastric juices earlier in the gastro-intestinal tract (GI tract). These gastric juices break food down for nutrient extraction. The full range of B-complex vitamins is required for your body to make sufficient hydrochloric acid to digest food. Most multivitamins contain a full range of B-complex vitamins to help in this regard.

Boost Your Bowels with Probiotics

As mentioned above, take a full-spectrum probiotic supplement on an empty stomach. I usually find first thing in the morning or in the evening before bed is best. Beneficial bacteria are needed in the intestines to manufacture essential nutrients like vitamin B12; ensure absorption of vitamins like B1, B2, B12, and vitamin K; keep harmful bacterial and yeast infections under control; and ensure proper absorption of nutrients in your food. Ideally, look for one that contains a variety of lactobacilli (L.) and bifidobacteria (B.), including *L. rhamnosus, L. plantarum, L. acidophilus, L. paracasei, L. salivarius, B. animalis lactis, B. bifidum, B. breve, B. infantis,* and *B. longum.*

Bulk Up to Reduce Toxins: Fiber and Flax

Bulking up your stool by eating more fibrous foods and taking fiber supplements causes toxins to bind to the fiber to be eliminated from the body. Although there are many fiber supplements on the market, they are not created equally. Ideally, add two tablespoons of freshly ground flax seeds into your daily diet. Not only is it an excellent fiber supplement, but it also boosts your intake of essential fatty acids, which are needed for healthy intestinal function.

Magnesium: Nature's Gentle Laxative

Magnesium is one of the best natural and gentle laxatives. It adds water to the stool to ensure that toxins are easily eliminated. Some experts estimate that up to 80 percent of the population is deficient in this important mineral that is essential to over five hundred bodily processes, so it is imperative to get more magnesium, particularly during the Colon Cleanse Weekend. Many of the Top Colon-Cleansing Foods above are also high in magnesium. In addition to the multivitamin, take 400mg daily of this mineral, ideally paired with calcium in equal proportions for best results. Because calcium and magnesium are synergistic, taking them together is best. Fortunately, many companies have developed calcium-magnesium formulations in a single capsule or tablet for convenience. Calcium citrate and magnesium citrate are the most absorbable forms of these minerals.

Herbal Intestinal Cleansers

There are literally dozens of great herbal intestinal cleansers, so picking only a few of the best was a challenge. Because herbs are a form of natural medicine, they need to be treated with respect. If you are pregnant or nursing, have a serious health condition, or are taking medication, consult a qualified health practitioner before using them. Make sure you choose someone knowledgeable about the thousands of studies that prove herb effectiveness because, unfortunately, this is not an area of expertise most physicians currently possess.

You don't need to purchase all of the herbs below—one to three is sufficient. I've included extras should you have difficulty finding the ones you want in your area. Most of these herbs are readily available in dried, capsule, or tincture (alcohol-extract) form; choose the form that is most convenient for you. If you have ever had a substance abuse problem or have impaired liver function, choose a format other than alcohol-based tinctures, for obvious reasons.

Aloe Vera (Aloe vera)

Aloe vera juice has been used for over four thousand years, and for good reason. It has the ability to heal ulcers and ulcerations in the digestive tract while also helping to stimulate elimination of fecal matter from the intestines. It is rich in amino acids, chlorophyll, enzymes, essential oils, vitamins, and minerals, as long as it is from a pure source. Drink a quarter cup of aloe vera juice, twice daily, preferably on an empty stomach. Note: aloe vera juice is not the same as the gel, which is more concentrated. Avoid using "aloes" or "aloe latex" or products containing them, as their eliminative action is quite strong. Also be aware that aloe vera products frequently contain sugar, preservatives, and other additions, all of which should be avoided on the Colon Cleanse Weekend.

Cascara Sagrada (Rhamnus purshiana DC)

Cascara sagrada is also known as sacred bark, perhaps for its ability to create movement where none previously existed. It both tones and cleanses the intestines, helping to eliminate built-up toxic matter. Because it also influences a process known as peristalsis, in which gentle spasms help to move the waste matter through the intestines, it is best to use only small doses of this potent herb. And you may wish to stay close to home during the Colon Cleanse Weekend, as this herb tends to increase the "call of nature." Use twenty drops of the alcohol extract three times daily. Alternatively, boil the herb: one-half teaspoon to one cup of water. It's best to make in medium- to large-sized batches so you won't go through this process three times daily. Bring to a boil then lower heat and let simmer, covered in a small pot, for one hour. Strain out the herb. Drink one-half cup of the remaining herbal tea three times daily.

Licorice Root (Glycyrrhiza glabra L.)

Although I am not talking about the candy, licorice, licorice root tea does taste a lot like the sweet that bears its name and sometimes contains this medicinal herb. Licorice root works on multiple levels to restore health to the intestines: it reduces inflammation, helps eliminate toxic waste, and soothes the intestinal walls. It also helps give the body a boost when it has been under a lot of stress, whether emotional or physical. Avoid using licorice root if you have high blood pressure, take heart medication, or have experienced kidney failure. Licorice root is readily available as a tincture (take one teaspoon three times daily) or in teabag form for convenience.

White Walnut (Juglans cinerea L.)

White walnut, also known as butternut or *Juglans cinerea* L., cleanses and tones the whole digestive tract, including the intestines. Additionally, it helps to kill undesirable pathogens that may exist in the bowels. It also helps heal the bowels' mucous membranes. Take one teaspoon of the alcohol extract three times daily. Alternatively, boil the dried herb in water (one teaspoon of the dried herb to one cup of pure water). Bring to a boil, and let simmer for one hour. Drink one-half cup three times daily.

THE EXERCISES

Colon-Cleansing Cardio

Exercise is important for intestinal health, as it helps keep toxins moving through the body until they are eliminated. During the next three days of the Colon Cleanse Weekend it is imperative to do some form of cardiovascular exercise.

You'll need to do at least twenty minutes a day. If you have been inactive prior to the detox, you may wish to do cardiovascular exercise for ten minutes twice each day. Whatever you choose, make sure it adds up to at least twenty minutes. Also be sure that it is sufficient to boost your heart rate without making you feel like your heart is going to jump out of your chest. It should never feel so intense that you cannot carry on a discussion with someone during activity.

You can choose any form of cardiovascular exercise you prefer, including brisk walking, jogging, stair climbing, cycling, spinning, or dancing. You don't need a health club membership or expensive equipment. You don't need special training or a body-hugging outfit to get fit. All you need is some motivation and a willingness to get moving. Pick a form of activity you will actually enjoy; I believe making exercise fun means you're more likely to do it.

Knees to Chest

Additionally, a yoga posture known as *Apanasana* is also helpful during intestinal cleansing to help keep toxins eliminated. It should be done at least once per day but can be done more often if you want. It is also known as *knees to chest*, which gives a fairly clear description of what it entails. Here is how you perform the knees to chest yoga posture.

Lie on your back with your legs extended. (See Figure 6.1.)

Bend your knees toward your chest, keeping your knees separated from each other and your hands resting on the floor. Point your feet, and keep your toes together. (See Figure 6.2.)

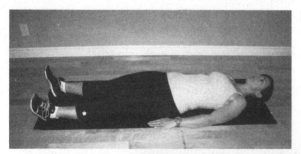

Figure 6.1

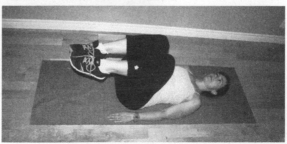

Figure 6.2

Next, draw your knees together and wrap your arms around your legs. Hold for at least twenty seconds. (See Figure 6.3.)

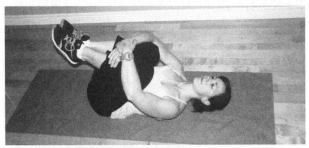

Figure 6.3

Gently roll toward your left side, and hold for at least twenty seconds. Then roll toward your right side, and hold for at least twenty seconds.

Repeat the process at least three times, then relax on your back with your legs extended. (See Figure 6.1.)

THE SPA TREATMENTS

Acupressure Abdominal Massage

My first experience with the gentle colon-cleansing power of acupressure abdominal massage came many years ago when I was seventeen as part of a visit to my naturopath, Dr. James D'Adamo, the now-famous doctor known as one of the innovators behind the Blood-Type Diet.

I wasn't really convinced that such a simple massage could help with my colon-cleansing efforts, but it did. So I encourage you to keep an open mind and a gentle-but-firm hand to perform the acupressure abdominal massage I've outlined here:

Start by laying on your back with your knees up and feet flat on the floor. You can be clothed during this massage.

Begin massaging at the lower part of your abdomen toward the right side of your body. Massage in gentle-but-firm clockwise

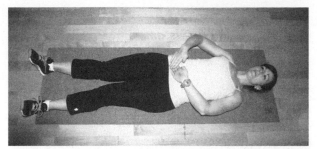

Figure 6.4

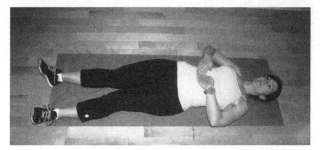

Figure 6.5

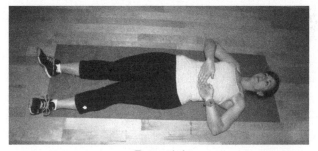

Figure 6.6

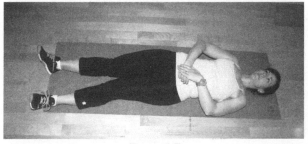

Figure 6.7

circles that slowly move upward along the right side of your abdomen. The heel of your hands works well, but you can use your fingertips if you find it easier.

Next, move across the upper part of your abdomen from right to left, continuing in gentle-but-firm clockwise circles.

Then continue the clockwise circles while gradually moving down the left side of your abdomen.

Continue massaging from the lower left side of your abdomen to the lower right side.

Repeat two more times. Perform this acupressure abdominal massage at least once daily for all three days of the Colon Cleanse Weekend. See Figures 6.4 to 6.7.

THE WEEKEND

By now you have a good understanding of the intestines and the valuable role they play in your overall health. You are also knowledgeable about the best foods, nutrients, herbs, exercises, and therapies that ensure a clean colon. I'll help you put together your whole weekend here.

I've outlined a step-by-step approach to the Colon Cleanse Weekend detox below. Of course, you can choose the foods from the list that appeal most to you. I don't want this to feel arduous or for you to feel deprived. Choose a wide variety of foods for the best results and to prevent boredom on the plan. It is important that you have a personalized plan that fits your health, budget, and schedule. The Colon Cleanse Weekend detox is designed to be flexible and individualized so you'll get the best results.

Here's what your three-day weekend will look like.

Days one to three:

Upon rising—Drink a large glass of water (two cups) with the fresh juice of one-half lemon. Alternatively, drink a large glass of warm water with the fresh juice of one-half lemon. Add a few drops of liquid stevia if you prefer a sweeter-tasting beverage. Wait twenty minutes before eating.

Breakfast—Be sure to include some of the colon-cleansing foods mentioned above. Some good options include Chia Breakfast Tapioca (page 266), Veggie Scramble (page 262), or cooked brown rice with almond milk.

Multivitamin

Optional nutrients

Herb (first dose of selected herbs)

Midmorning—Colon Cleanse Herbal Tea (page 246) or Super-Detoxifying Green Tea Lemonade (page 243)

Snack, such as an apple with almond butter, raw unsalted walnuts, the Heirloom Tomato and Basil Salad (page 257), or celery sticks with almond butter or Herbes de Provence Cashew Cheese (page 250)

Exercise—colon-cleansing cardio, knees to chest

Lunch—Weekend Wonder Detox Signature Salad (page 258) or other large detoxifying salad, with garbanzo beans and pumpkin seeds on top

Cucumber Mint Refresh (page 240) or a smoothie with almond milk, berries, and freshly ground flax seeds

Vitamin C

Optional nutrients

Herb (second dose of selected herbs)

Midafternoon—Large glass of warm water (with lemon juice), a cup of Colon Cleanse Herbal Tea (page 246), or Citrus Boost (page 241)

Snack, such as apple with almond butter, raw unsalted walnuts, roasted squash with flax oil, or celery sticks with Herbes de Provence Cashew Cheese (page 250)

Acupressure abdominal massage

Dinner—Lentil Bowl (page 263) with Lemon-Garlic Greens (page 252) or Roasted Red Pepper Chickpea Mash (page 263) and sautéed kale and red peppers or Curried Garbanzo Bean and Squash Stew (page 265)

Fresh cup of Colon Cleanse Herbal Tea (page 246), Watermelon Ice (page 241), or Honey-Turmeric Tea (page 247)

Herb (third dose of selected herb)

After dinner—Bowl of berries, Cantaloupe Ice (page 241), or Citrus Boost (page 241)

Before bed—Take some quiet time to turn off the television. Find a quiet place to sit, close your eyes, and take some deep breaths.

Write in the Colon Cleanse Weekend Detox Journal (at the end of this chapter).

CONCLUDING THE
COLON CLEANSE WEEKEND

Well done! You've completed the Colon Cleanse Weekend. You are likely feeling lighter and cleaner. Your whole body will thank you.

After the Colon Cleanse Weekend you may wish to keep incorporating foods, nutrients, herbs, exercises, or spa treatments into your day-to-day life. I encourage you to do so. Clean intestines are integral to all aspects of your health, so just maintaining good health in this area can make a difference to your overall health too.

You may choose to do the Colon Cleanse Weekend every weekend for a month or one weekend out of every month. The choice is yours. You know your lifestyle and schedule best, so choose the option that works best for you.

If you continue to follow the Colon Cleanse Weekend for longer periods, every three weeks just take one week off from any herbs and concentrated fiber supplements you're using so they don't become habit forming.

You may also wish to try some of the other health-building weekend detoxes I've included throughout *Weekend Wonder Detox*. I often recommend that people start with the Colon Cleanse Weekend and, once the bowels seem to be moving well, do the Lymphomania Weekend, followed by the Love Your Liver Weekend. But there are no rules here—do whatever feels best for you.

THE WORKSHEETS

The Grocery List

For easy Colon Cleanse Weekend prep, print this list and take it with you when you go to your local health food and grocery stores. Remember that not all of the items are essential. Purchase only the foods, nutrients, herbs, and items for the spa treatments you've selected.

Foods

Below you'll find many intestinal-cleansing foods with which to stock your fridge and pantry. Also, make sure your pantry is stocked with the essential items you learned about in Chapter 2 for any recipes you select.

Top Intestinal-Cleansing Foods (remember, you're trying to get the fiber count up to thirty-five grams each day). You don't need to purchase all of these items, just the ones you prefer, although I encourage you to stretch your horizons a bit.

acorn squash	butternut squash
adzuki beans	cashews
almonds	chia seeds
amaranth	collard greens
beet greens	currants (red or white)
black beans	elderberries
black turtle beans	flax seeds
blackberries	French beans
blueberries	garbanzo beans (chickpeas)
boysenberries	gooseberries
Brazil nuts	hemp seeds
broad beans (fava)	hubbard squash
brown rice	kale
buckwheat groats	kidney beans

lentils

lima beans

loganberries

millet

mung beans

mustard greens

navy beans

oats (gluten-free)

pine nuts

pinto beans

pistachios

pumpkin seeds

quinoa

raspberries

sesame seeds

spaghetti squash

spinach

strawberries

summer squash

sunflower seeds

Swiss chard

teff

turnip greens

walnuts

white beans

wild rice

yellow beans

zucchini squash

Nutritional Supplements

multivitamin and mineral (essential)

probiotics (essential)

magnesium (optional but highly recommended)

Herbs Selected

Choose one to three of the following herbs:

aloe vera juice

Cascara sagrada

licorice root

white walnut

The Colon Cleanse Weekend Detox Journal

You may wish to print off a copy of the journal page to make it easier to complete.

Energy: Rate your energy (from 0 to 10, with 0 meaning complete exhaustion, and 10 meaning abundant energy). Before the detox _____ After the detox _____

Pain: Rate your pain levels (from 0 to 10, with 0 meaning none, and 10 meaning unbearable, constant pain). Before the detox _____ After the detox _____

Mood: Rate your mood (from 0 to 10, with 0 meaning extremely moody, depressed, angry, or irritable, and 10 meaning extremely happy). Before the detox _____ After the detox _____

Weight: Before the detox _____ After the detox _____

Checklist of Intestinal-Cleansing Foods Consumed

Try to eat at least thirty-five grams of fiber daily. Here is a quick chart of the Top Intestinal-Cleansing Foods with the number of grams of fiber listed beside each. Calculate your daily totals, and write down the amount of fiber you consumed each of the three days here.

	Day 1	Day 2	Day 3
daily fiber totals	_____	_____	_____

Legumes

adzuki beans (one cup cooked) 17

black beans (one cup cooked) 15

black turtle beans (one cup cooked) 17

broad beans (fava) (one cup cooked) 9

French beans (one cup cooked) 17

garbanzo beans (chickpeas) (one cup cooked) 12

kidney beans (one cup cooked) 16

lentils (one cup cooked) 16

lima beans (one cup cooked) 14

mung beans (one cup cooked) 15

navy beans (one cup cooked) 19

pinto beans (one cup cooked) 15

white beans (small) (one cup cooked) 19

yellow beans (one cup cooked) 18

Nuts

almonds (one ounce) 4

Brazil nuts (one ounce) 12

cashews (one ounce) 1

pine nuts (one ounce) 12

pistachios (one ounce) 3

walnuts (one ounce) 2

Seeds

chia seeds (two tablespoons) 10

flax seeds (two tablespoons) 4

hemp seeds (two tablespoons) 2

pumpkin seeds (one-half cup) 3

sunflower seeds (one-quarter cup) 3

sesame seeds (one-quarter cup) 4

Berries

blackberries (one cup, fresh or frozen) 8

blueberries (one cup, fresh or frozen) 4

boysenberries (one cup, fresh or frozen) 7

currants (red or white) (one cup, fresh or frozen) 5

elderberries (one cup, fresh or frozen) 10

gooseberries (one cup, fresh or frozen) 6

loganberries (one cup, fresh or frozen) 8

raspberries (one cup, fresh or frozen) 8

strawberries (one cup, fresh or frozen) 3

Grains

amaranth (one cup cooked) 6

brown rice (one cup cooked) 4

buckwheat groats (one cup cooked) 5

millet (one cup cooked) 2

oats (gluten-free, one-half cup cooked) 4

quinoa (one cup cooked) 5

teff (dry, uncooked) (one-quarter cup cooked) 6

wild rice (one cup cooked) 3

Leafy greens

beet greens (one cup cooked) 4

collard greens (one cup cooked) 5

kale (one cup cooked) 2.6

mustard greens (one cup cooked) 5

spinach (one cup cooked) 4

Swiss chard (one cup cooked) 4

turnip greens (one cup cooked) 5

Squash

acorn squash (one cup cooked) 9

butternut squash (one cup cooked) 6

hubbard squash (one cup cooked) 7

spaghetti squash (one cup cooked) 2

summer squash (one cup cooked) 5

zucchini squash (one cup cooked) 3

Selected Nutrients

Be sure to take the multivitamin each day. Write down any additional nutrients you've opted to take throughout the detox. Remember that you don't need to take all of them. Check off each day you take them.

	Day 1	Day 2	Day 3
multivitamin and mineral	_____	_____	_____
probiotics	_____	_____	_____
magnesium (optional)	_____	_____	_____

Selected Herbs

Indicate the one to three herbs you've selected to take throughout the detox. Check off each day you take them. Most herbs need to be taken three times daily.

	Day 1	Day 2	Day 3
aloe vera juice	_____	_____	_____
Cascara sagrada	_____	_____	_____
licorice root	_____	_____	_____
white walnut	_____	_____	_____

Exercises

Check off each time you complete the exercises in the Colon Cleanse Weekend. Make sure to do both exercises daily.

	Day 1	Day 2	Day 3
colon-cleansing cardio	_____	_____	_____
knees to chest	_____	_____	_____

Selected Spa Treatment

Check off each time you complete the colon-cleansing spa treatment. Make sure you do it every day.

	Day 1	Day 2	Day 3
acupressure abdominal massage	_____	_____	_____

Observations and Thoughts

Day 1: _____
_____
_____
_____

Day 2: _____
_____
_____
_____

Day 3: _____
_____
_____
_____

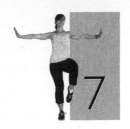

THE SKIN
REJUVENATION
WEEKEND

BENEFITS OF DETOXIFYING YOUR SKIN

- Fewer acne breakouts
- Fewer rashes or hives
- Clearer skin
- Softer, smoother skin
- Less dry skin
- Reduced risk of psoriasis or eczema

Most people know that beauty is more than skin deep, but our social emphasis on physical appearance can make even the most flawless-skinned beauty self-conscious. Not surprisingly, anyone suffering from skin problems may be even more self-conscious. With some help from foods, water, and herbs, all as part of the Skin Rejuvenation Weekend, along with a healthy dose of self-appreciation, it is possible to not only love the skin you are in but also improve its health and appearance as well.

You are what you eat, but you are also what you put on your skin. Not only is the skin the body's largest organ; it is the body's largest detoxification organ. Your skin also prevents your body from becoming dried out or waterlogged when you've been exposed to water, and it helps to protect your body from elements, temperature variation, microorganisms, sun damage, and other items. Your skin may show toxic overload, stress, hormonal imbalances, and nutritional deficiencies. By working on the internal causes of skin concerns, the results are more effective than just applying a cream or ointment and hoping for the best.

JULIA BEATS BREAKOUTS

Julia M. came to see me concerned about her sensitive skin and her tendency toward breakouts with hives, rashes, and occasional bouts of acne. The skin issues were taking their toll on her self-esteem, and she didn't want to keep slathering cortisone creams on them. Although these creams had once made the skin condition look improved, they no longer made a difference. Besides that, she had read an article on the Internet about the long-term immune system and other problems linked to cortisone cream use, and it just didn't sit well with her.

I explained that the skin is often a reflection of other aspects of health and symptoms. For instance, hives and rashes tend to reflect sensitivity to toxins in the environment, particularly those that come in contact with the skin such as fabric softeners, laundry detergents, and personal care products.

Upon further investigation Julia reported that she used commonly available brands of laundry soaps and fabric softeners. She couldn't believe the number of toxic ingredients they contained. Like most people, Julia assumed that because these products were readily available, they must be safe. We evaluated the products she used for personal care—soap, moisturizers, bug repellents, perfumes, and so forth. She was using many

continues

continued

common products full of petrochemical byproducts, synthetic fragrances, and artificial colors and preservatives. I asked her to switch to completely natural products. She agreed and asked me whether it would be alright to make the switch over the course of a month to consider her budgetary constraints. I encouraged her to take the time she needed to make the changes, explaining that it was more important that she stick to the changes for the long term.

Julia also agreed to eliminate many of the toxin-containing processed, packaged, and prepared foods as she prepared for her Skin Rejuvenation Weekend later in the month (once she had made the switch to more natural personal care and laundry products).

One month later Julia came to see me looking excited and eager to tell me something. She explained that, after she made the switch to more natural laundry and personal care products and doing the Skin Rejuvenation Weekend detox, the rashes and hives stopped. Her acne was significantly improved as well.

She was so thrilled to have clearer skin and fewer breakouts that she decided to stick with the natural products and eat more of the healthy foods. Periodically she does the Skin Rejuvenation Weekend as "general maintenance," as she described it.

Once you learn more about your skin's needs and experience the Skin Rejuvenation Weekend you'll understand why Julia M. felt changed from her skin detoxification experience and why she no longer looks at her skin in the same way.

WHY SHOULD I DETOXIFY MY SKIN?

Most of what you slather on your skin will be absorbed directly into your bloodstream, where it will have access to your brain and other organs. This is why carefully selecting the skin care and body care products you use is so important. Most of these products (yes, even the brand-name and highly priced ones) are full of toxic in-gredients that should never be put on skin. When you slather on creams full of petroleum products (most are!), synthetic preserva-tives, and other toxic ingredients, these ingredients quickly gain access to your blood.

Organs like the liver and kidneys will become involved in getting rid of these harmful toxins, but these organs can become overwhelmed if we keep throwing more toxins at them.

The skin also purges internal toxins through perspiration. When we clog our pores with personal care products we reduce what our bodies are able to eliminate through sweat. And al-though that doesn't sound like a big deal, sweating is one of the best detoxification mechanisms your body has at its disposal. This is particularly true of heavy metals like mercury, lead, and cad-mium, all of which our bodies are exposed to in day-to-day life. Heavy metals are often best eliminated from the body through the skin, so blocking the skin's ability to do so can cause toxic buildup in seemingly unrelated parts of the body.

The Skin Rejuvenation Weekend is different from the other detoxes in *Weekend Wonder Detox* for a couple of reasons. The obvious one is the focus on the skin instead of another organ, but this detox also focuses on internal cleansing as well as the detox-ification of personal care products that can be absorbed through the skin and impede its ability to detoxify. So you'll eat foods and use natural supplements, herbs, and therapies that cleanse your skin from the inside, but you'll also give your beauty care and per-sonal care products an overhaul too. The latter means that you'll significantly reduce the quantity of toxins to which you are ex-posed in the future, giving your skin a better opportunity to heal and a reduced chance of experiencing skin issues.

SIGNS OF STRESSED-OUT SKIN

There are many signs that your skin is overloaded with harmful toxins. They range from acne breakouts to eczema or psoriasis.

SIGNS YOU WOULD BENEFIT FROM A SKIN DETOX

Here are some of the symptoms and conditions that are linked to excessive toxic load for the skin:

acne, blackheads, or whiteheads	eczema
blotchy or ruddy skin	hives
dry and/or flaky skin	psoriasis
dry, scaly patches of skin	rashes

When Beauty Turns Ugly

As you learned in Chapter 1, there are more than 850 toxins lurking in most of the common cosmetics and personal care products. Most of my clients are amazed at how much better their skin looks and feels after they switch to more natural skin care products. The very product you may be using to improve your skin may actually contribute to skin conditions and toxic overload in your body.

The first way to detox your personal care products is to read the labels. If there is no ingredient list on the label, the company most likely has something to hide, so avoid these products altogether. If there is an ingredient list, be sure to check for ingredients like the toxic ones I mentioned earlier, including parabens—butyl-, ethyl-, isobutyl-, methyl-, and propyl-parabens; butylene glycol; numbered dyes like yellow dye #5 and red dye #4; petrolatum; fragrance; benzoates; sodium lauryl sulphate; diethanolamine (DEA) and ethanolamine (TEA); imidazolidinyl urea and diazolidinyl urea; PVP/VA copolymer; stearalkonium chloride; dioxin; fluoride; coal tar; and lead (rarely listed but found in lipsticks—be sure it says "lead-free").

I'm not asking you to eliminate all your favorite products if you don't want to. Use them if you want to, but know the risks. But on the Skin Rejuvenation Weekend it is imperative to give your skin a break from all these toxic ingredients. You can switch to more natural options found in the health food store—just be sure to read the labels, because many of the personal care products in health food stores still contain some toxic ingredients. And check out the healthy natural options in the Recipes section at the back of this book for recipes to make your own personal care products. Most of these products are simple to make and much purer than anything you'll find in the stores.

THE DIET

You'll be eating a very simple diet over the next few days on the Skin Rejuvenation Weekend. For some reason many people immediately assume that means bland and boring food, but that couldn't be further from the truth. There are lots of delicious foods in the Recipes section at the back of this book to help you eat delicious and nutritious food. The diet for this weekend includes six Skin Rejuvenation Weekend essentials and the Top Fourteen Skin-Cleansing Foods.

The Skin Rejuvenation Weekend Program Essentials

1. **One of the most critical components of healthy skin is water.** The body is made up of approximately 80 percent water and needs its stores replenished. Every cell in the body is dependent on water for good health, including skin cells. Water helps keep the skin properly hydrated. Although the need for water varies from person to person, I find that during a detox people benefit from drinking one-half quart or one-half liter (almost the same amount) for every fifty pounds of weight they're carrying, up to about three quarts or liters. I know this is a lot of water, and you may feel like you're spending your weekend in the bathroom, but your body needs water to flush out toxins. Without sufficient water, toxins can become absorbed back into the bloodstream. Fresh vegetable and fruit juices count toward your total amount of water. Vegetable juices are preferable to water because they contain water along with plentiful amounts of vitamins, minerals, phytonutrients, and

enzymes. Freshly made fruit juices also contain these beneficial substances but tend to be high in sugars, so they are best consumed in minimal amounts. And if you drink caffeinated or alcoholic beverages, which are not part of the Skin Rejuvenation Weekend (with the exception of green tea), then add two additional cups of water for every cup of coffee, tea, or alcohol you drink.

2. **Give your skin an oil change.** Healthy skin requires plenty of health-boosting essential fats like Omega 3s, yet most people don't get enough of them. Flax, chia, hemp, walnuts, and fatty fish like wild salmon, mackerel, and sardines tend to have high levels of Omega 3s. Because Omega 3 fats are sensitive to heat, choose cold-pressed flax seed or hempseed oil and raw, unsalted walnuts that have been stored in the refrigerator section of your natural food store. Eat a handful or two, minimum, of raw nuts and seeds daily throughout the detox. You can also eat fatty fish daily if you'd like, but that's not a requirement.

3. **Drink two to three cups of freshly made vegetable juices daily throughout the detox.** Juices like carrot, cucumber, celery, or other vegetable juices can be helpful at cleansing the skin from the inside while also providing plenty of nutrients to help build healthy skin cells. It's great if you have a juicer, but you don't need one to make fresh vegetable juices, particularly if you have a powerful blender. Cucumber is easily broken down into juice in a typical blender, and this is fortunate because it is also the best skin-cleansing vegetable.

4. **If you're particularly vulnerable to acne, you'll need to completely avoid many of the acne-triggering foods.** Fortunately, you may already be avoiding most of these foods because they are not good for a detox. Some of the culprits are alcohol, coffee, eggs, meat, milk, wheat, sugar, tea, iodized salt (and foods that contain it), and vinegar. Tobacco and some medications and hormones also cause acne. If that sounds like the bulk of your diet, don't worry—there are lots of great food options left, which you will soon discover.

5. **Eliminate toxic oils.** Hydrogenated fats (margarine, short-ening, lard, or products made with them, such as cookies, pies,

packaged foods, buns, pizza, etc.) and fried foods (French fries, onion rings, potato chips, nachos, hamburgers, etc.) or foods containing oils that have been excessively heated are not included in the Skin Rejuvenation Weekend. Also, avoid "vegetable oil," "safflower oil," "canola oil," and "sunflower oil" found in most grocery stores. Most grocery store oils have been heated excessively during processing even before they reach the shelves. Most canola oil is genetically modified and therefore not a suitable food product. Extra-virgin olive oil is an excellent choice for cooking on low to medium temperatures. Be careful not to let it smoke, as that is an indicator the oil has changed molecular structure and will now cause inflammation in the body. Cold-pressed oils found in most health food stores are also a healthy choice. Flax oil is great but shouldn't be heated or used for cooking.

6. **Nonorganic meat and poultry contains hormones, sugar, and antibiotics, all of which increase your body's toxic load.** In addition, many people are sensitive to the hormones and other chemicals in meat. Skin problems can be an indication of a sensitivity or allergy. Switch to organic meat and poultry.

7. **Reduce your toxin exposure in personal care products.** If you use chemical-laden skin and hair care products, your body cannot rely on its largest detoxification organ to eliminate toxins. Instead, your skin is working in reverse, absorbing more poisons into your cells. Switch to natural hair and skin care products that are free of fragrances, colors, or other synthetic chemicals that have a tendency to irritate skin as well as increase your body's toxic load. Refer to the section above that indicates many of the common toxins you'll need to avoid. Refer to Chapter 1 for a reminder of the health problems linked to these common toxins.

Top Fourteen Skin-Cleansing Foods

There are many great skin-cleansing foods, but the following fourteen are some of the best. Be sure to eat at least three of these foods every day of the Skin Rejuvenation Weekend. Of course, you can eat more, and I encourage it. The more of these foods you incorporate into your daily diet, the healthier your skin will be.

Almonds—An excellent source of protein, fiber, B-complex vitamins, vitamin E, calcium, iron, magnesium, and zinc, almonds help to eliminate toxins and improve the elasticity as well as repair skin from the inside out.

Avocado—Most people think that avocados are unhealthy due to their high fat content, but this couldn't be further from the truth. Avocados are rich in vitamin E, which your body needs to keep skin soft and healthy. They are also high in betasitosterol, which is valuable to protect against skin cancer and other cancers. Rich in monounsaturated fat, avocado helps keep the skin moisturized. Avocados help heal acne, sun damage, and wounds. Avocados are also rich in vitamin D, which is essential for healthy skin.

Blueberries—Rich in antioxidants that reduce free radical damage, blueberries also prevent the breakdown of collagen in the skin, which is needed to prevent wrinkling. Blueberries' proanthocyanidins also help heal sun-damaged skin.

Cantaloupe—The orange color is the giveaway that this fruit is high in beta carotene, the precursor of vitamin A in the body. Vitamin A is essential for clear skin, free of blemishes.

Cucumbers—Cucumbers were highly popular in many ancient civilizations, including Egypt, Greece, and Rome, thanks to their skin-healing properties. They are particularly beneficial to rehydrate skin from the inside out, but they can also be mashed and applied to affected areas of skin, left on for up to an hour to help heal dermatitis or any skin irritation.

Fish and sea vegetables (Fatty kinds like wild salmon, mackerel, anchovies, or sardines)—Fish is rich in Omega 3 fatty acids eicosapentanoic acid (EPA) and docosahexanoic acid (DHA) that decrease inflammation and improve skin conditions like psoriasis, dry skin, and inflamed skin. Sea vegetables are also a good source of DHA. You can use nori sheets to wrap brown or black rice and vegetables. You can also use hijiki, which typically comes in thin, spaghetti-like strands, or kelp, both of which can be rehydrated by soaking in water. Either hijiki or kelp make a great addition to soup. There are many types of seaweed available in health food stores, so don't be afraid to experiment. There are even kelp noodles, which are naturally gluten-free and a delicious, mineral-rich, low-carb alternative to high-carb pastas. Kelp noodles are found in the refrigerator section of most health food stores, whereas other types of seaweed are dried and packaged.

Flax—Rich in Omega 3 fatty acids and vitamin E, flax seeds help skin stay moist and blemish-free. They also reduce inflammatory skin conditions like psoriasis and moisturize dry skin from the inside out. Add one tablespoon of cold-pressed flax oil to smoothies or sprinkle two tablespoons of flax seeds on your food each day to benefit from their skin-soothing properties.

Leafy greens—Rich in many nutrients like vitamin K, which helps heal wounds, and chlorophyll, which gives these veggies their green color and improves blood and skin health, leafy greens are an excellent choice on the Skin Rejuvenation Weekend.

Pumpkin and pumpkin seeds—Like cantaloupe and sweet potatoes, pumpkin is also rich in beta carotene, the precursor to vitamin A. As a result it helps with healing and protecting against sun damage as well as helps scars fade and wounds heal. Raw, unsalted pumpkin seeds are packed with skin-healing Omega 3 fatty acids and should be eaten daily for best results.

Squash—High in beta carotene, which helps protect the skin from UV damage, squash is an excellent skin-cleansing superfood.

Strawberries—Rich in the antioxidant superoxide dismutase and its partner nutrient, manganese, strawberries help eliminate free radicals and improve some skin conditions. However, some people with eczema or psoriasis are sensitive to strawberries, so if you have one of these conditions, you may want to watch your strawberry intake.

Sunflower seeds—Rich in protein, zinc, Omega 6 fatty acids, and vitamin E, sunflower seeds are highly beneficial to the skin. They help heal rough, dry, or flaky skin as well as improve the condition of eczema.

Sweet potatoes—Thanks to their high amounts of carotenes, like beta carotene, sweet potatoes are delicious and help heal skin conditions. Avoid adding sweeteners to these already sweet-tasting veggies. Sweet potatoes are also rich in other antioxidants like vitamin C, which helps eliminate infections, including from the skin's surface.

Walnuts—Rich in skin-softening and healing Omega 3 fatty acids, walnuts are a great addition to your diet if you want to improve your skin. Eat only raw, unsalted walnuts that have been stored in a refrigerator because these oils go rancid quickly.

Some people may wonder why papayas, which are rich in carotenes and enzymes, are not on the list. Because some papayas have been genetically modified, I don't recommend using them unless you are sure of their organic status.

By increasing your consumption of water, fruits, and vegetables, particularly those listed above, your body will begin to cleanse. Some people may find that their skin temporarily worsens as they start a cleansing program. If that is the case, it usually lasts for a day or two and then improves. That's a sign that toxins are being eliminated via the skin. Usually the skin clears up fairly quickly.

THE SUPPLEMENTS

There are many great nutritional supplements and herbs that assist with skin cleansing. Of course, you don't need to take all of them—just two or three is fine. Read the following section to learn which one(s) might be best suited for your particular needs. And as always be sure to follow the dosage recommendations to maximize the benefits of your cleanse.

Critical Skin-Cleansing Nutrients

Many different nutrients play critical roles in skin health. To help prevent any deficiencies, be sure to take a high-quality multivitamin and mineral. Select one that is devoid of additives, colors, preservatives, gluten, and common allergens like corn, soy, and wheat. You may wish to take additional nutrients that are beneficial to the skin. Here are some of the essential skin health nutrients.

Eliminate dry skin with vitamin A—A vitamin A deficiency can be a primary cause of dry skin. Supplement with 10,000 IU of vitamin A daily. Don't take higher levels of vitamin A unless you are working with a qualified nutritionist, as excessive amounts can build up in the body.

Improve skin health with vitamin D3—Vitamin D3 is essential for great skin health. Although it is called a vitamin, it functions more like hormones in the body and helps to ensure a strong and healthy immune system. Vitamin D3 is available in drops, which is the easiest way to take it. I suggest 2,000 IU (which usually works out to be two drops of vitamin D3 in liquid form) daily during the Skin Rejuvenation Weekend, but because deficiencies can take longer to address, it's advisable to continue this dose afterward.

Protect skin with vitamin E—Vitamin E is really a combination of several different compounds known as alpha-, beta-, delta-, and gamma-tocopherol and alpha-, beta-, delta-, and gamma-tocotrienol. I know it sounds more like a sorority than a collection of nutrients, but these nutrients are so powerful that some experts estimate that we could reduce health care costs in the United States by $8 billion if people took adequate vitamin E supplements.[1] That's because vitamin E is involved in so many health functions and is imperative to good health. It is a powerful free radical scavenger that protects skin against aging and wrinkling. It also has anticancer properties, helps protect against skin cancer, helps reduce scar formation, and speeds wound healing. It can be applied directly onto the skin in areas where there are concerns, such as scars, wrinkles, rashes, and breakouts, but it is also advisable to take a natural-source combination of tocopherols like those mentioned above. Make sure it is in the "D" form, not "DL" form, which is synthetic. Studies that show vitamin E is not beneficial or, worse, harmful usually use the latter synthetic form. So the label should read "D-alpha tocopherol," *not* "DL-alpha tocopherol." Take 400 IU of vitamin E daily.

Moisturize skin with Omega 3 fatty acids—Insufficient essential fatty acids can also be a causative factor for dry skin, particularly an Omega 3 fatty acid deficiency. Cold-pressed flax oil found in the refrigerator section of most health food stores is an excellent choice. Add one to two tablespoons to your salads or in smoothies, or supplement with three to six capsules daily depending on their size and manufacturer's directions. Never heat this oil.

Eliminate skin-damaging free radicals with zinc—This mineral plays a critical role in the functioning of an important antioxidant enzyme called superoxide dismutase (SOD). SOD is one of the body's best defenses against aging and wrinkling as well as many diseases. Zinc is also important for burn and wound healing. Although it is found in many types of sprouts, pumpkin seeds, onions, sunflower seeds, nuts, dark leafy green vegetables, beets or beet greens, carrots, and peas, many people still have a deficiency that requires higher amounts to address. I encourage you to eat these foods on a regular basis while supplementing with zinc gluconate or zinc citrate, which are the superior forms of this mineral due to their ability to be readily absorbed by the body. Skin problems indicate a need for a higher dosage than common recommendations; I suggest a daily dose of 30mg on the Skin Rejuvenation Weekend unless you're working with a skilled nutritionist. Because zinc can build up to toxicity levels, it is important not to take high doses for more than a few months.

More Skin-Cleansing Nutrients

The main nutrients that support healthy skin include chromium, potassium, zinc, essential fatty acids, and vitamins A, B-complex, C, D3, and E. You'll get most, if not all, of these nutrients in a multivitamin and mineral supplement. Remember to check the product label to ensure you are getting sufficient amounts of vitamins A, D3, E, and zinc, without getting amounts higher than those recommended above, particularly if you're taking a multiple along with other supplements. Exceeding recommended doses can be easy when combining multis with single nutrients. For example, you might have 5,000 IU of vitamin A in your multi and take another 10,000 IU in a vitamin A supplement, totaling 15,000 IU, which is higher than the recommended amount.

Herbal Skin Cleansers

Herbs are naturally powerful healers. Although there are many great skin-cleansing and healing herbs, the ones I like best are yellow dock and cleavers. I've also included dong quai and black cohosh for women who experience hormonally linked skin issues, either premenstrually, perimenopausally (the decade before menopause), and menopausally. You don't need to take all of the herbs below—just one or two is fine. Both are readily available from most health food stores in dried, capsule, or tincture (alcohol-extract) form. If you have any liver impairment or a history of alcoholism, I advise against using tincture form.

I've listed the scientific name of each herb so you'll be sure to obtain the correct one when purchasing it. Some herbs have similar common names.

Yellow Dock (Rumex crispus)

Yellow dock is great for skin conditions, particularly psoriasis or acne, but it has beneficial properties that would help many other skin concerns. A new study in the journal *Nutrition Research and Practice* found that yellow dock is a potent antioxidant and has anticancer activity, making it a good choice if you've had sun-damaged skin. Use one to two teaspoons of dried herb per cup of water. Bring to a boil, then cover and reduce heat for one hour. Remove from heat. Strain and drink one cup three times daily. Alternatively, take a quarter to half teaspoon of tincture three times a day.

Cleavers (Galium aperine)

Drinking cleavers tea three times daily can help with skin problems and reduce acne flare-ups. It is also good for the kidneys and lymphatic system, so you'll be helping to cleanse your body of toxins on multiple levels. This herb also goes by the name goosegrass or grip grass. Use two to three teaspoons of dried herb per cup of water. Let steep for twenty minutes. Then drink three cups daily.

Dong Quai (Angelica sinensis)

If your skin problems coincide with your menstrual periods, hormonal imbalances may be at fault. Dong quai is an excellent choice for women suffering from hormone imbalances. Although it can be made into a tea, I find the taste rather disgusting and tend to recommend it in capsule form (follow package instructions) or as a tincture (one teaspoon three times daily).

Black Cohosh (Actaea racemosa)

If you suspect that your skin problems, particularly dry skin, are hormonally linked and if you are in the decade prior to menopause (usually forty to fifty), which is known as perimenopause, or if you are currently menopausal or postmenopausal, you might benefit from taking black cohosh. It is an excellent hormone-balancing herb; however, be sure to choose a high-quality one. Take one teaspoon of the tincture three times daily. If you are perimenopausal, menopausal, or postmenopausal, it is also important that you avoid caffeine and alcohol (with the exception of the amount in the tincture) and engage in regular exercise to help balance hormones. Avoid using if you are pregnant or lactating.

THE EXERCISE

Cardio to Heal the Skin

Exercise is important for skin health, as it one of the primary outlets for toxin elimination. Additionally, it boosts blood (and, therefore, oxygen, which is carried in the blood) to the surface of the skin to help keep it healthy. Oxygen is also great for killing harmful bacteria and fungi that are linked to skin infections and other conditions.

During the next three days of the Skin Rejuvenation Weekend it is imperative to do some form of cardiovascular exercise. You'll need to do at least twenty minutes a day. If you have been inactive prior to the detox, you may wish to do cardiovascular exercise for ten minutes, twice each day. Whatever you choose, make sure it adds up to at least twenty minutes. Also be sure that it is sufficient to boost your heart rate without making you feel like your heart is going to jump out of your chest. It should never feel so intense that you cannot carry on a discussion with someone during activity.

You can choose any form of cardiovascular exercise you prefer, including brisk walking, jogging, stair climbing, cycling, spinning, or dancing. You don't need a health club membership or expensive equipment. You don't need special training or a body-hugging outfit to get fit. All you need is some motivation and a willingness to get moving. Pick a form of activity you will actually enjoy; making exercise fun means you're more likely to do it. Furthermore, body-hugging, synthetic fabrics can actually prevent proper elimination of toxins and cause bacterial buildup on the skin's surface. So if possible, try wearing cotton, bamboo, or other natural clothing. If your skin is quite sensitive, you might prefer organic cotton because regular cotton is heavily sprayed with pesticides. Don't assume or listen to salespeople who tell you synthetic fabrics are superior—they are not. Most synthetic fabrics are made from petroleum products. Yes, that oil and gas that can't be used in your car could actually be in your clothing, another possible culprit for skin conditions.

Ideally, it is best to get outside for a brisk walk or hike in nature, where you can breathe fresh, oxygen-rich air. Of course, you'll want to be sure that you are protected from the sun if you are outside. That doesn't mean slathering your skin with a toxic sunscreen (most are!). Instead, either wear a long-sleeve shirt or pants and a hat or choose a natural, fragrance-free, paraben-free, and color- and preservative-free sunscreen from your local health food store. Most sunscreens sold in drug and grocery stores are full of toxic ingredients and have even been linked with skin cancer.

THE SPA TREATMENT

When it comes to the skin, there are so many wonderful spa treatments that can help heal blemishes, reduce dryness, and lessen the appearance of wrinkles. However, the treatments depend on the quality of ingredients used. Some spas may claim the products used in their treatments are "all natural," yet this is rarely the case. I've been told this and reviewed the products only to find cancer-causing parabens and colors, among other toxic ingredients, on the list. Choosing products free of toxic ingredients is important; otherwise, you will defeat all of your best efforts.

The Aromatherapy Skin Softener Bath
(Bath Option One)

Who doesn't love a relaxing, warm bath? Why not make your next bath also healing for your skin? It's easier than you think. Simply adding some pH-balancing baking soda to the water along with some pure, high-quality, skin-healing essential oils can transform your next bath into a healing oasis. Ideally, it's best if you can take a minute or two to dry skin brush beforehand. You can learn more about dry skin brushing on page 108. Choose one bath daily during the Skin Rejuvenation Weekend. If you don't have a bathtub, that's okay—just choose some of the other spa treatments below.

Fill a bath with hot (but not too hot, as this dries out the skin and can be exhausting) water.

Add one-half cup baking soda.

Add five or six drops of pure, high-quality essential oils of lavender, geranium, or chamomile. (You can use all three or just one—whichever you prefer.) It's best to add the oils directly under the faucet while the bath water is still running to help them disperse throughout the water. Always do a twenty-four- to forty-eight-hour skin test on the inside of your arm to be sure you have no allergic reactions to the oils. Although pure essential oils are highly safe and therapeutic, it is possible to have the occasional person who has an allergic reaction to something that normally heals the skin.

Relax in the bath for about twenty minutes. The baking soda and essential oils will soften your skin, help eliminate any microbes that may be on the surface of your skin, and soothe any inflamed areas.

Always drink a large glass of water after your bath.

At-Home Thalassotherapy Bath
(Bath Option Two)

Many spas offer seaweed treatments to improve skin and assist with weight loss. The latter may seem particularly surprising to most people, but there is some solid research supporting its weight-loss supporting properties. The benefits of seaweed skin treatments (called thalassotherapy) are largely linked to seaweed's rich mineral and nutrient composition.

You will need:

One-quarter cup dried seaweed (it really doesn't matter which type you use, as all types of seaweed are rich in nutrients, but choose one that has been ground or grind it yourself in a small coffee grinder). You can use for the bath the same seaweed you eat, but some health food stores carry preground seaweed created especially for bathing.

One-half cup hot water

Three drops of pure lavender essential oil

Mix the seaweed and hot water together and let sit for five minutes.

Add the seaweed mixture to your bath, and add the lavender under the running water to encourage it to disperse throughout the bath.

Soak for at least twenty minutes.

Always drink a large glass of water after your bath.

Note: You may want to use a small sieve in your bathtub to catch any seaweed solids before they go down the drain, particularly if you plan to use this bath regularly.

The Salt Body Scrub

The salt body scrub is an excellent way to improve circulation in your skin, and this further promotes healing. The unrefined sea salt is full of skin-healing minerals, the essential oils eliminate harmful microbes and alleviate blemishes, and the olive oil helps moisturize the skin.

You will need:

Twenty to thirty drops of pure, high-quality essential oils of lavender or peppermint (depending on personal preference—lavender is relaxing, and peppermint is invigorating).

One-quarter cup extra-virgin olive oil

One-half cup finely ground, unrefined sea salt (it has a natural grayish color due to the many minerals it contains)

Place the essential oils in a small bowl with the extra-virgin olive oil and mix together. Add the sea salt, and mix together.

On damp skin, scrub your skin with a handful of the scrub, working upward from the feet toward the heart, and again from the hands, toward the heart. Rinse and pat skin dry.

Skin Clarity Facial

This simple facial is made with fresh food ingredients to nourish your skin. It is simple to make at home and is beneficial for all skin types. The cucumber has natural antiseptic qualities, enzymes to remove dead skin, and minerals to nourish skin. The avocado contains protein for healthy skin along with essential fats to improve skin texture and plump up fine lines. The honey is a natural antiseptic that kills harmful bacteria. Be sure to choose unpasteurized honey. Mix together:

Two-inch piece of cucumber

One-half avocado

One teaspoon of honey

Mash or grind all the ingredients together. A food processor works well for this purpose. Smooth over your face, neck, shoulders, or any "trouble spots" on your skin. Relax and allow to sit on the skin for twenty minutes. Rinse with warm water. Use this facial daily throughout the Skin Rejuvenation Weekend.

THE WEEKEND

By now you have a good understanding of the skin and the valuable role it plays in ensuring toxins are eliminated from your body. You are also knowledgeable about the best foods, nutrients, herbs, exercises, and therapies that ensure a healthy skin. I'll help you put together your whole weekend here.

I've outlined a step-by-step approach to the Skin Rejuvenation Weekend detox below. Of course, you can choose the foods from the list that appeal most to you. I don't want this to feel arduous or for you to feel deprived. Choose a wide variety of foods for the best results and to prevent boredom on the plan.

It is important you have a personalized plan that fits your health, budget, and schedule. The Skin Rejuvenation Weekend detox is designed to be flexible and individualized so you'll get the best results.

Here's what your three-day weekend will look like.

Days one to three:

Upon rising—Drink a large glass of water (two cups) with the fresh juice of one lemon. Add a few drops of liquid stevia if you prefer a sweeter-tasting beverage. Wait twenty minutes before eating.

Cardio to heal the skin

Salt body scrub

Breakfast—Be sure to include some of the skin-rejuvenating foods mentioned above. Some good options include half a cantaloupe with fresh blueberries or an almond milk-avocado-strawberry smoothie, Veggie Scramble topped with pumpkin and sunflower seeds (page 262), or cooked brown rice topped with almond milk, strawberries, and blueberries, and Skin Rejuvenation Herbal Tea (page 247).

Multivitamin

Optional nutrients

Herb (first dose of selected herbs)

Midmorning—Large glass of water (with lemon if desired), a cup of Skin Rejuvenation Herbal Tea (page 247), or Super-Detoxifying Green Tea Lemonade (page 243)

Snack, such as fresh or frozen (slightly thawed) blueberries, raw unsalted walnuts, and sunflower and pumpkin seeds

Lunch—Weekend Wonder Detox Signature Salad (page 193) or other large detoxifying salad topped with roasted squash, walnuts, pumpkin seeds, sunflower seeds, blueberries, and a tablespoon of flax seed oil

Citrus Boost (page 241) or Skin Rejuvenation Herbal Tea (page 247)

Vitamin C

Optional nutrients

Herb (second dose of selected herbs)

Midafternoon—Large glass of water (with lemon if desired), a cup of Skin Rejuvenation Herbal Tea (page 247), or Cucumber Mint Refresh (page 240)

Snack, such as raw unsalted walnuts, pumpkin seeds, or sunflower seeds, celery sticks with almond butter

Dinner—Salmon Parcels (page 266) with Lemon-Garlic Greens (page 252) or Ginger Chili Quinoa (page 264) and Chili Lime Green Beans (page 252)

Fresh cup of Celery Cucumber Juice (page 240), Skin Rejuvenation Herbal Tea (page 247), Honey-Turmeric Tea (page 247), or Carrot Celery Juice (page 240)

Herb (third dose of selected herb)

After dinner—Colon Cleanse Herbal Tea (page 246) or Cantaloupe Ice (page 241)

Skin clarity facial

Aromatherapy skin softener bath or at-home thalassotherapy bath

Before bed—Take some quiet time to turn off the television. Find a quiet place to sit, close your eyes, and take some deep breaths.

Write in the Skin Rejuvenation Weekend Detox Journal (at the end of this chapter).

CONCLUDING THE SKIN REJUVENATION WEEKEND

You just completed the Skin Rejuvenation Weekend. Your skin texture is likely improved, some blemishes have disappeared, and you may have that healthy glow many of my clients report. Your skin may look improved, but your whole body will thank you for taking the time to pay attention to its needs.

After the Skin Rejuvenation Weekend you may wish to keep incorporating foods, nutrients, herbs, exercises, or spa treatments into your day-to-day life. You may also wish to keep switching your personal care products, clothing, and laundry detergents to more natural and healthful options. Of course, I encourage you to do so. Healthy skin that isn't absorbing toxins is essential to a healthy body.

You may choose to do the Skin Rejuvenation Weekend every weekend for a month or one weekend out of every month. Or if you've had serious skin issues, you may want to stick with it for a full month. The choice is yours. You know your lifestyle and schedule best, so choose the option that works best for you.

If you continue to follow the Skin Rejuvenation Weekend for longer periods, just take one week off every three weeks from any herbs so they don't become habit forming and your body doesn't adapt too much to them.

You may also wish to try some of the other health-building weekend detoxes I've included throughout *Weekend Wonder Detox*. I often recommend that people with skin issues start with the Colon Cleanse Weekend and, once the bowels seem to be moving well, do the Lymphomania Weekend, followed by the Love Your Liver Weekend. But there are no rules here—do whatever feels best for you.

THE WORKSHEETS

The Grocery List

For easy Skin Rejuvenation Weekend prep, print this list and take it with you when you go to your local health food and grocery stores. Remember that not all of the items are essential. Purchase only the foods, nutrients, herbs, and items for the spa treatments you've selected.

Foods

Here are the skin rejuvenation foods you'll need. Also, make sure your pantry is stocked with the essential items you learned in Chapter 2 and for any recipes you select.

— almonds
— avocados
— blueberries
— cantaloupe
— cucumbers
— fish
— flax seeds and flax seed oil
— leafy greens
— pumpkin and pumpkin seeds
— strawberries
— sunflower seeds
— sweet potatoes
— walnuts

Nutritional Supplements

— multivitamin and mineral (essential)
— vitamin A (essential but is often included in sufficient amounts in the multivitamin)
— vitamin D (essential but is often included in multivitamins)
— vitamin E (essential but is often included in multivitamins)

— Omega 3s (essential, may say "DHA-EPA" or "Fish oil" on the package)

— zinc (optional but is often included in sufficient amounts in the multivitamin)

Herbs Selected

Choose one to three of the following herbs:

— yellow dock

— cleavers

— dong quai (optional if you get premenstrual skin flare-ups)

— black cohosh (optional if your dry or irritated skin is linked to perimenopause, menopause, or postmenopause)

Optional Items if You Selected the
Aromatherapy Skin Softener Bath

— baking soda

— essential oils (one is fine but you can blend all three if you prefer): lavender, chamomile, and/or geranium

Optional Items if You Selected the
Salt Body Scrub

— lavender or peppermint (depending on personal preference) essential oil

— extra-virgin olive oil

— unrefined sea salt

Skin Clarity Facial

— one cucumber

— one avocado

— raw, unpasteurized honey

The Skin Rejuvenation Weekend Detox Journal

You may wish to print off a copy of the journal page to make it easier to complete.

Energy: Rate your energy (from 0 to 10, with 0 meaning complete exhaustion, and 10 meaning abundant energy). Before the detox _____ After the detox _____

Pain: Rate your pain levels (from 0 to 10, with 0 meaning none, and 10 meaning unbearable, constant pain). Before the detox _____ After the detox _____

Mood: Rate your mood (from 0 to 10, with 0 meaning extremely moody, depressed, angry, or irritable, and 10 meaning extremely happy). Before the detox _____ After the detox _____

Weight: Before the detox _____ After the detox _____

Checklist of Skin-Rejuvenating Foods Consumed

Try to eat at least five a day. Check the ones you ate each day.

	Day 1	Day 2	Day 3
almonds	_____	_____	_____
avocado	_____	_____	_____
blueberries	_____	_____	_____
cantaloupe	_____	_____	_____
cucumber	_____	_____	_____
fish	_____	_____	_____
flax seeds and flax seed oil	_____	_____	_____
leafy greens	_____	_____	_____
pumpkin and pumpkin seeds	_____	_____	_____
squash	_____	_____	_____
strawberries	_____	_____	_____
sunflower seeds	_____	_____	_____
sweet potatoes	_____	_____	_____
walnuts	_____	_____	_____

Selected Nutrients

Be sure to take the multivitamin and vitamin C each day. Write down any additional nutrients you've opted to take throughout the detox. Remember that you don't need to take all of them. Check off each day you take them.

	Day 1	Day 2	Day 3
multivitamin and mineral	_____	_____	_____
vitamin A	_____	_____	_____
vitamin D3	_____	_____	_____
vitamin E	_____	_____	_____
Omega 3 fatty acids	_____	_____	_____
zinc	_____	_____	_____

Selected Herbs

Indicate the one to three herbs you've selected to take throughout the detox. Check off each day you take them. Most herbs need to be taken three times daily.

	Day 1	Day 2	Day 3
black cohosh	_____	_____	_____
cleavers	_____	_____	_____
dong quai	_____	_____	_____
yellow dock	_____	_____	_____

Exercise

Check off each time you complete cardiovascular exercise. Make sure to do it every day.

	Day 1	Day 2	Day 3
cardiovascular exercise	_____	_____	_____

Selected Spa Treatment(s)

Check off each time you complete the skin-rejuvenating spa treatments. It's not necessary to do all of them, but whichever one(s) you choose, make sure you do it every day.

	Day 1	Day 2	Day 3
aromatherapy skin softener bath	_____	_____	_____
at-home thalassotherapy bath	_____	_____	_____
salt body scrub	_____	_____	_____
skin clarity facial	_____	_____	_____

Observations and Thoughts:

Day 1: _____

_____

_____

_____

Day 2: _____

_____

_____

_____

Day 3: _____

_____

_____

_____

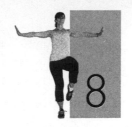

8

THE FAT BLAST
WEEKEND

BENEFITS OF THE FAT BLAST WEEKEND
• Weight loss • Less tissue puffiness • Fat reduction • Less bloating • Flatter abdomen

Most people want a quick and effective way to get started losing those extra pounds, and the Fat Blast Weekend is a terrific solution. Unlike other detoxes in *Weekend Wonder Detox*, we're not really targeting a specific organ to correct any imbalances in this detox, so you'll find that this chapter and, therefore, detox is a bit different from the others.

In this weekend we'll be targeting fat stores and amping up your metabolism. Of course, if you're quite heavy, one weekend is not going to cause you to lose all the extra weight you may have gained over years; however, it will help you to get a jump on healthier eating and exercise as well as help you drop a size and up to six pounds. Everyone is different, so your results may vary from the next person.

The Fat Blast Weekend is not an excuse to live unhealthily the rest of your life. It is not an excuse to eat anything and everything every other day of the week. Instead, it is a quick way to get results and a great way to begin a healthier lifestyle.

After you've completed the Fat Blast Weekend you may want to just keep it going every day or every weekend as part of your overall healthy eating and exercise regime. You may also benefit from periodically doing a Love Your Liver Weekend because the liver helps with weight loss and fat breakdown, making these two weekend detoxes a perfect pair.

JOANNE DROPS A DRESS SIZE

Joanne M. had always been what she described as "a bit chubby," but when she hit her forties the weight just seemed to be piling up. She'd "tried everything," she told me when she came to see me about her weight issues. Normally I'm skeptical when someone tells me they've tried everything, but, when Joanne and I reviewed the plans she'd actually tried, there were a whole lot—high protein, low carb, and just about everything in between. Instead of getting results, she just lost confidence in herself and felt like a failure.

I asked her to try to forget everything she ever did to lose weight; after all, most of the diet plans out there are just gimmicks someone created with no nutritional knowledge (even most MDs never study a single nutrition course!) and certainly not based in scientific research. She agreed to commit to transforming her weight by starting with a single long weekend. I outlined the foods to avoid, foods to eat, fat-blasting supplements, and herbal remedies. Then we explored exercise and some spa treatments that not only feel like pampering but also target fat to help mobilize it for elimination. All of these items are based on well over two decades of research I've conducted to help people with stubborn weight lose it for good.

Joanne came back in several days explaining that she "followed the Fat Blast Weekend to the letter." She glowingly reported that she had

continues

continued

dropped five pounds and was down a dress size. She confessed that she really hadn't expected ANY results because of her previous experiences. She also asked me whether there were any problems continuing the Fat Blast Weekend for longer periods of time. I explained that it was fine, as it was created to work in harmony with the body's organs and organ systems, not to overburden them the way many popular diets do.

She continued to avoid all the junk foods she previously ate and told me she was actually really enjoying the taste of the healthier food. She stayed on the herbal tea and supplements as well and kept eating many of the Super Fat-Blasting Foods. Despite all this success, however, Joanne was still having trouble with exercise. I explained that sometimes any exercise may feel intense but that it should feel like a challenge, not a hardship. Most people simply choose exercise that is tedious, boring, or downright awful. When I asked her whether there was ever a sport or activity that she enjoyed, she shared that she used to love mountain biking and agreed that she would love to start it again.

Joanne added monthly Love Your Liver Weekends and periodic full-blown Fat Blast Weekends to her new dietary and exercise habits, along with monthly follow-up appointments. I am thrilled to report that Joanne lost fifty-three pounds in the year after she started the Fat-Blast Weekend. She has a new lease on life and loves every minute of the confidence she built by eating better and getting back to a sport she loves.

THE DIET

Let's explore the dietary component of the Fat Blast Weekend. It's important that you follow the dietary suggestions as closely as possible. Remember, it's just three days for now. Like Joanne, you can always continue the diet afterward, but right now you just need to follow the suggestions for the weekend. That feels less daunting for most people.

Here are twelve Fat Blast Weekend essentials to follow.

1. **Avoid the Top Ten Foods That Make You Fat.** Some foods actually sabotage your best weight-loss efforts. For this weekend detox avoiding them is essential. If avoiding these foods for only three days is not possible for you, then you may have a food addiction that needs to be addressed. Usually that means you may be eating some food in an effort to satisfy an emotional need in your life. Some reflection may be necessary to get to the bottom of these types of food addictions. The Top Ten Foods That Make You Fat include ice cream, corn and tortilla chips, pizza, French fries, potato chips, bacon, hot dogs, doughnuts, soda, and diet soda. For a more detailed explanation of these foods and how they make you fat, see below.

2. **Drink at least three cups of fresh vegetable juices daily.** You can buy an inexpensive juicer; there are many excellent ones under $50. Alternatively, watch for one at a local garage sale, because they regularly seem to find their way to the curb. For the purpose of weight loss, it is imperative to keep all sugars to a minimum, including fruit sugars (more on this below). It's easy to make your own juices using high-water vegetables that include carrots, celery, cucumber, peppers, and tomatoes. Tomatoes can be blended in a blender, so they do not require a juicer at all. Check out some of my favorite fat-blasting juice recipes at the back of this book.

3. **Snack at least twice daily between meals.** Healthy fat-busting snacks are the key here, as they help stabilize your blood sugar levels. Roller-coaster blood sugar levels cause weight gain and fat hoarding in your body; you simply cannot lose weight without balancing your blood sugar. Snacks that help with blood sugar balancing should include some protein (learn more about this topic in item six below), fiber, and vegetables. There are lots of great snack options in the Recipes section at the back of this book, but here are a few to help get your creative juices flowing: celery sticks with almond butter and topped with pumpkin seeds, raw sunflower seeds and carrot sticks, black bean dip with vegetable crudités, cooked quinoa with chopped veggies, or an almond or coconut milk smoothie.

4. **Drink water.** Although the need for water varies from person to person, I find that during a detox people benefit from drinking one-half quart or one-half liter (almost the same amount) for every fifty pounds of weight you're carrying, up to about three quarts or liters. I know this is a lot of water, and you may feel like you're spending your weekend in the bathroom, but your body needs water to flush out toxins. Without sufficient, toxins can become absorbed back into the bloodstream. Fresh vegetable and fruit juices count toward your total amount of water. Vegetable juices are preferable to water because they contain water along with plentiful amounts of vitamins, minerals, phytonutrients, and enzymes. Freshly made fruit juices also contain these beneficial substances but tend to be high in sugars, so they are best consumed in minimal amounts. And if you drink caffeinated or alcoholic beverages, which are not recommended on the Fat Blast Weekend (with the exception of green tea), then add two additional cups of water for every cup of coffee, tea, or alcohol you drink.

Ideally, filtered, alkaline water is best. That doesn't necessarily mean an expensive water filtration unit, however; even a $15 water stick can help alkalize your water. See the Resources section at the back of this book for more information. If you don't have access to alkaline water, completing the detox is still okay—just be sure to drink at least ten cups of water daily.

5. **Eat at least one large salad daily.** Before you cringe at the idea of eating salad let me explain that your salads should be anything but boring. If it's boring, you're not doing it right. Your salad should be a powerhouse of flavor. A fat-blasting salad should take only minutes to prepare and will greatly assist your weight-loss efforts. I've included a Fat-Blasting Salad chart below (see page 256) to help guide you further.

6. **Eat a high-protein food at every meal and as a snack.** Eating a high-protein food at every meal or snack helps to regulate your blood sugar levels, and this is critical for weight loss. That doesn't mean eating lots of meat, as doing so will stress the kidneys and intestinal tracts and can lead to acid buildup in the joints. It doesn't

necessarily mean eating meat at all, although you can have small amounts of lean chicken, turkey, eggs, or fish if you'd like. If you choose chicken, turkey, or eggs, be sure it is organic, and eat only six ounces maximum once daily—that's smaller than the size of a deck of cards. You can also select many great vegetarian protein foods, including almond slices or raw almonds, black beans, Brazil nuts (raw, unsalted), cashews (raw, unsalted), chickpeas, edamame (organic only), flax seeds (ground), Great Northern beans, hempseeds (ground), kidney beans, lentils, lima beans, macadamia nuts (raw, unsalted), mung bean sprouts, navy beans, pecans (raw, unsalted), pinto beans, pistachios (raw, unsalted), pumpkin seeds, quinoa (cooked), romano beans, sesame seeds, sunflower seeds (raw, unsalted), tofu (organic only), and walnuts (raw, unsalted).

7. **Avoid all sugars, natural or otherwise, and avoid all synthetic sweeteners.** Only stevia that doesn't contain fillers and other ingredients is acceptable. If you're not sure whether you can handle this guideline, remember that you only need to do it for three days, so it's the perfect way to break a sugar addiction. The digestive systems of most people who are overweight are incapable of handling the amount of sugars and carbohydrates they eat. Additionally, most people, heavy or thin, are addicted to sugars. When it comes to weight loss, natural sugars like honey, maple syrup, agave nectar, and others aren't much better than their white-sugary counterparts. For the Fat Blast Weekend avoid all fruit except lemons for your water and no more than half an apple in each vegetable juice if you need it for palatability (up to a maximum of one and a half daily).

8. **Take a high-quality multivitamin and mineral supplement to ensure you address possible deficiencies.** To burn fat, your body needs many nutrients, so supplying them throughout the weekend is important. Of course, it is fine to continue taking them afterward. Be sure to choose a brand that is free of colors, preservatives, sugars, synthetic sweeteners (sucralose and aspartame are synthetic sweeteners that should be avoided on the Fat Blast Weekend), and other artificial ingredients and fillers.

9. **Eat small meals and snacks frequently throughout the day, and eat only until you feel comfortably full.** Most people overeat, thinking that they are not yet "full." They've equated full with a heavy, bloated feeling, which it isn't, causing them to continue eating. Pay attention to how you feel, and stop eating earlier than you normally do. You can always have a juice or a snack later if you're still hungry, but it is important to reeducate your body about healthy food portions.

10. **Ditch the dairy.** Forget what you've heard about so-called research proving the fat-burning effects of dairy products. Dairy products simply aren't the health or weight-loss foods most people believe them to be. Many of these types of studies have been biased due to their funding sources. Besides that, the people who report on them often make giant leaps in assumptions. For example, there is excellent research showing that diets high in calcium help people lose weight. The assumption here is that milk is high in calcium, so it must be the ideal weight-loss food. But milk and dairy products are acid forming in the body, bog down the lymphatic system (read more in Chapter 4, "The Lymphomania Weekend"), and require large amounts of enzymes to digest properly. Cow's milk is for baby cows, not humans. Modern commercialization processes also ensure that cow's milk and other dairy products are full of antibiotics that throw off the healthy bacterial balance in your bowels (which leads to weight gain!), hormones that plump up cows (and humans), and genetically modified ingredients (which cause health problems in humans).

11. **Eat at least five of the Top Eight Fat-Blasting Foods daily.** They include almonds, apple cider vinegar, avocado, chiles, cinnamon, coconut (unsweetened only), coconut oil, flax seeds, flax seed oil, grapefruit, green tea, legumes (beans), leafy greens (kale, mustard greens, spinach, spring mix, and other leafy greens), lemons (or lemon juice), olive oil (cold-pressed, extra-virgin), seaweed, tomatoes, turmeric, walnuts, and wild salmon.

12. **Avoid eating for at least three hours before bedtime.** During sleep your body busily absorbs the nutrients from the food

you ate earlier in the day and goes to work repairing cells and tissues. If this period is bogged down with digestion, which consumes vast amounts of your body's energy, there is insufficient energy left to perform these other important tasks, many of which are critical to weight loss. So stop eating before bed. If you absolutely need something, drink water or a vegetable juice, or snack on some raw veggies.

Top Ten Foods That Make You Fat

I have worked in the field of health and nutrition for over two decades. I have advised thousands of people on ways to improve their eating habits, make healthy food choices, lose weight, and feel great. After more than twenty years it still astounds me when someone who claims to be following my advice tells me that it doesn't work and that they have not experienced any benefits, ranging from weight loss to increased energy. Inevitably, I ask them some questions about what they ate in the past weekend and—surprise, surprise—we find that they are not following my program. They think they are, but somehow some of the worst foods you can consume find their way into meals and snacks throughout the weekend.

No one eats a perfect diet. I believe it is impossible with the amount of processed, packaged, and prepared "foods" in the grocery stores as well as the nutrient-deficient fruits and vegetables harvested through industrial growing methods or genetic modification. Despite these challenges, we can still do our best to feed our bodies the healthiest foods we can find. If we do this on a daily basis, it is not so harmful to sneak in a less-than-perfect snack once in a while (i.e., maybe once a week). If it becomes a daily habit, however, all your efforts to eat healthy the rest of the time will not make a difference to your weight-loss efforts.

Here are the worst foods you can eat at any time, and especially if you are trying to lose weight. They are listed from "dire" to "disastrous."

10. **Ice cream.** I once had a client justify his ice cream habit by saying it was a good source of calcium. Nice try, but the majority of ice creams sold in stores, ice cream parlors, and restaurants is loaded with sugar, trans fats, and chemicals to give it flavor and color. These artificial ingredients are often chemicals known to damage the brain and nervous systems. You may think, *That sounds bad, but what does it have to do with losing weight?* The brain is a delicate organ that controls, among other things, our metabolic processes. Chemicals that interfere with the brain can throw our metabolism out of balance, affecting our capacity to lose weight.

9. **Corn chips and tortilla chips.** I love Mexican food and dipping chips into great-tasting salsa and guacamole. Unfortunately, the most common type of tortilla chip is made of genetically modified (GM) corn, one of the most common GM crops grown today. Even organic corn is high in sugar, which contributes to blood sugar fluctuations and can lead to fat hoarding and, ultimately, weight gain. Rapid blood sugar fluctuations can make us moody or irritable. Tortilla chips tend to be fried in high-production facilities where the oil is already rancid from both overheating and age. These bad oils can also cause inflammation in the body.

8. **Pizza.** Although not all pizza contributes to weight gain, most does. That's largely due to the refined white flour crust and artificial ingredients such as trans fats and dough conditioners. The white flour acts just like sugar, which causes blood sugar fluctuations and fat hoarding in your body. And as you learned earlier, cheese, like other dairy products, is not the health food most people claim it is; instead, it is high in saturated fats and heavily processed, causing it to be a burden to an already burdened body.

7. **French fries.** No matter how you slice it (the potato, in this case), there is no such thing as a nutritious French fry. Most fries are consumed at fast-food restaurants and, as the name implies, fried in various types of overused and overheated oils. Much like tortilla chips above, these oils are rancid and contribute to the excessive levels of trans fats found in fried foods. The high temperatures required to fry potatoes also contribute to the formation of

acrylamide, a highly carcinogenic substance that also contributes to inflammation in the body. Studies are demonstrating that inflammation is not only linked to cancer but also to arthritis, heart disease, and weight gain. Avoid the fast-food drive-thru, and eliminate the temptation to order fries with your meals. If you make meals at home, get rid of the deep-fryer and remove the packaged, frozen, oven-baked fries from your grocery list as well.

6. **Potato chips.** After reading about French fries, it seems redundant to add potato chips to the list. These easily accessible snacks can be a serious craving for even the most health-conscious eaters. Health Canada researchers have found that chips have even higher levels of acrylamide than French fries. In fact, out of the foods tested, potato chips had the highest level of this toxin.

5. **Bacon.** Bacon has been a staple in many breakfasts and sandwiches for decades, and it seems to be experiencing a troubling renaissance as an ingredient in everything from sweets to main courses. Although all those celebrity chefs on the food channels joke about how bacon is not a health food and then proceed to add it to just about every recipe, bacon consumption is no laughing matter. The journal *Circulation* published research illustrating that daily consumption of bacon and other processed meats can increase the risk of diabetes by 19 percent and the risk of heart disease by a whopping 42 percent.

A study from the University of Columbia found that consuming bacon fourteen times a month—less than once every two days—significantly increased the risk of lung disease and reduced lung function. If you ever come across a weight-loss program that includes bacon—and they are out there—avoid it at all costs. No reputable health professional would ever claim bacon is part of a healthy eating plan, considering the level of fat, salt, and nitrites it contains.

4. **Hot dogs.** Like other processed meats, hot dogs contain high levels of sodium nitrites, a carcinogen that has been linked to brain tumors in infants and leukemia in children. A University of Hawaii study concluded that eating hot dogs and other processed meats increased the risk of pancreatic cancer by 67 percent.[1]

3. **Doughnuts.** Here is one of those snack foods that seems to be part of the troubling "bacon on everything" trend. Doughnuts are often 35 to 40 percent trans fats. These are the worst kind of fats to eat at any time and especially if you are trying to cleanse your body or lose weight. The average doughnut also contains three hundred calories, toxic white sugar, artificial dough conditioners, and food additives.

2. **Soda.** An entire chapter of this book can be devoted to the damage soda will do to your body. A single can of regular soda will sidetrack your entire weekend detox efforts in multiple ways. In research reported by Dr. Joseph Mercola, on average a single serving contains ten teaspoons of sugar, 150 calories, 30 to 55mg of caffeine, and high levels of artificial food colors and sulphites.[2]

1. **Diet soda.** If you think diet soda is a good alternative beverage during your weekend detox, think again. Diet soda earns the top spot among the top ten foods that make you fat. It also earns bragging rights as the worst food of all time, and, like soda, I find it difficult to even refer to diet soda as "food." Take the worst features of regular soda, above, and then add artificial sweeteners like aspartame, which now goes by the catchy trade name of AminoSweet. The list of health conditions linked to aspartame and other artificial sweeteners is long and growing. They include anxiety attacks, birth defects, epilepsy, learning disabilities, migraines, reproductive problems, and depression.

Aspartame is even linked to sugar cravings and binge eating! That certainly won't help you on your weekend detox or at any other point in your life. If you are consulting with a professional who recommends these beverages as part of a healthy diet, you may want to reconsider your options for advice. I have worked with many people who lost weight and increased their energy and vitality after they eliminated diet soda.

Top Eight Fat-Blasting Foods

Tired of that spare tire? Sick of your love handles? You can increase your body's fat-burning power by eating more fat-blasting foods. There are many fabulous foods that fight fat, but the ones below are some of my favorites.

Leafy greens—Spinach, spring mix, mustard greens, and other dark leafy greens are good sources of fiber and powerhouses of nutrition. Research demonstrates that their high concentration of vitamins and antioxidants helps prevent hunger while protecting you from heart disease, cancer, cataracts, and memory loss.

Beans and legumes—Legumes are the best source of fiber of any foods. They help to stabilize blood sugar while keeping you regular. They are also high in potassium, a critical mineral that reduces dehydration and the risk of high blood pressure and stroke. A legume, soy is particularly good for fat burning. Isoflavones found in soy foods speed the breakdown of stored fat. In one study those who consumed high amounts of soy products shed three times more superfluous weight than did their counterparts who ate no soy.

Garlic and onions—This dynamic duo of foods contains phytochemicals that break down fatty deposits in the body while also breaking down cholesterol; killing viruses, bacteria, and fungi; and protecting against heart disease. With a little help from garlic and onions, you can burn fat while warding off illness.

Green tea—Study after study proves that drinking green tea dramatically reduces weight. It contains the phytonutrient epigallocatechin gallate (EGCG). EGCG increases the rate at which fat is burned in your body. Research at Tufts University indicates that EGCG, like other catechins, activates fat-burning genes in the abdomen to speed weight loss by 77 percent. Most studies show that drinking at least three cups daily offers the best health benefits.

Cayenne—This hot spice lessens the risk of excess insulin in the body by speeding metabolism and lowering blood glucose (sugar) levels before the excess insulin can result in fat stores. Spice up your next meal with cayenne, and shrink those love handles.

Turmeric—The popular spice used primarily in Indian cooking contains the highest known source of beta carotene, the antioxidant that helps protect the liver from free-radical damage. Turmeric also helps strengthen your liver while helping your body metabolize fats by decreasing the fat storage rate in liver cells. Add a teaspoon of turmeric into your next curry dish to help your body fight fat.

Cinnamon—Researchers at the US Department of Agriculture showed that a quarter to one teaspoon of cinnamon with food helps metabolize sugar up to twenty times better than food not eaten with cinnamon. Excess sugar in the blood can lead to fat storage, so before you sip that chai tea latte or eat your oatmeal, sprinkle on the cinnamon.

Flax seeds and flax seed oil—These seeds and oil attract oil-soluble toxins that become lodged in the fatty tissues of the body. Once attracted, they help to escort fat-soluble toxins out. That spells fewer fat stores and a trimmer you.

Note: See the Recipes section for instructions to "Create Health-Building Gourmet Salads in Minutes" and "Ways to Turn Your Salad into a Fat-Blasting Salad."

THE SUPPLEMENTS

Take a Multi to Avoid Deficiencies

Even a single vitamin or mineral deficiency can throw off the delicate balance of biochemical processes that determine the rate and efficiency at which your body burns (or stores) fat. That's why it is important to address any possible deficiencies by taking a multi throughout the Fat Blast Weekend, but you'll probably want to continue even after that. Be sure to choose one free of colors, fillers, and other synthetic ingredients. Many health food stores offer some excellent options.

Critical Nutrients for Fat Blasting

There are many nutrients that help burn fat and break down fat stores in your body. I've selected some of the best because I don't want you popping huge handfuls of pills. Carnitine and a

high-quality multivitamin are essential. Resveratrol with isoflavones and grape seed extract are optional.

Burn Fat Fast with Carnitine

If ever there were a fairy godmother who could grant wishes to lose
weight and increase energy, carnitine would be her name. Carnitine is a natural nutrient that burns fat to create more energy in
the body. And research proves its effectiveness. It transports fat to
the mitochondria (your cells' energy centers and fat incinerators)
to burn it as fuel, thereby creating energy. It sounds too good to
be true, but it is nutritional science at its best. In a recent study
people were divided into two groups—those who ate a healthy
diet and exercised moderately, and those who ate healthily, exercised, and also supplemented with two grams of carnitine daily.
The participants who supplemented with carnitine lost an average
of eleven pounds in twelve weeks, while those who ate well and
exercised lost only one pound in the same period.[3]

Most people obtain only about 50mg of carnitine in their daily
diet, which is insufficient to benefit from its weight-loss potential.
To burn fat you'll need to supplement with at least 500mg, but
some people don't notice the difference until they take 2,000mg
daily. Carnitine tartrate seems to yield the best results, as it is the
purest form of this nutrient. Take it on an empty stomach early in
the day—before breakfast is ideal. As an added bonus, you'll also
benefit from carnitine's ability to clear arteries, lower triglycerides
(when high), raise good HDL cholesterol, and protect the heart.

Make Fat Cells Self-Destruct with
Resveratrol and Isoflavones (optional)

What if you could take two nutrients that cause fat cells to self-
destruct? Well, you can. There are two phytonutrients (plant nutrients) discovered by Dr. MaryAnne Della-Fera at the University
of Georgia that literally cause fat cells to self-destruct. But that's
not all she discovered. She found that the nutrients resveratrol
and isoflavones, when taken together, reduce the cells' ability to
store fat by 130 percent and then cause them to disintegrate at a

246 percent faster rate than normal. Resveratrol is a natural substance found in grapes, and isoflavones are primarily found in soy foods. In Dr. Della-Fera's study people lost between four and ten pounds per week.[4] She obtained her results when people supplemented with 100mg each of resveratrol and isoflavones. Start with 100mg of each phytonutrient daily, and cut back to 25mg each if you experience nausea. Of course, for even better results, you can continue to take these supplements after the Fat Blast Weekend is over. Although these phytonutrients are often sold on their own, some stores sell them in a combination supplement.

Break Down Belly Fat with Grape Seed Extract (optional)

Grape seed extract is proven to stop the formation of belly fat. According to the study published in the journal *Molecular Nutrition and Food Research*, animals that were given the supplement grape seed extract built up less abdominal fat than animals who did not receive the supplement. According to the scientists, animals given grape seed extract also had a 61 percent increase in adiponectin, which is a hormone that speeds the conversion of fat into energy. The human equivalent of the dose used in the study would be 200mg of grape seed extract daily. This supplement will help stop your body from adding belly fat while encouraging it to break down abdominal fat stores into energy. Be sure to choose a high-quality grape seed extract because inferior ones use chemical solvents to extract the therapeutic benefits from grape seeds. You may be wondering whether you can get the benefit from wine. The answer is no. As for grapes, although you can blend grapes with seeds for a drink that contains grape seed extract, this juice is too high in sugar while you are trying to lose weight. It's a better option as you get closer to reaching your target weight.

Shrink Fat Cells with Conjugated Linoleic Acid (CLA) Combined with Chromium

Research at the University of Texas found that supplementing with the natural mineral chromium daily doubles fat loss without causing muscle loss.[5] There are different types of the mineral chromium, but the one with the best fat-burning effects is chromium glucose-tolerance factor, or chromium GTF. This is the form of chromium that is especially involved in balancing blood sugar levels, and this likely accounts for its weight-loss benefits. Supplement with just 200 to 500 MICROgrams daily. Scientists at the University of Texas also found that the benefits of chromium supplementation are superior when combined with conjugated linoleic acid (CLA). Supplement with two to three grams (2,000 to 3,000mg) of CLA daily for best results.

There are many other excellent natural supplements that help boost fat loss; however, they should never be taken in place of a healthy diet and exercise program. To learn more natural fat-burning supplements, check out my book 60 *Seconds to Slim*.

Herbs That Burn Fat

As always, Mother Nature provides great herbal remedies for weight loss. They are readily available in most health food stores. Green tea and saffron are two of the best fat burners.

Green Tea

Research at Tufts University indicates that EGCG in green tea, like other catechins, activate fat-burning genes in the abdomen to speed weight loss by 77 percent. You can drink green tea (as mentioned earlier) or you can take EGCG supplements if you prefer. EGCG also improves insulin use in the body to prevent blood sugar spikes and crashes that can result in fatigue, irritability, and cravings for unhealthy foods. Follow package instructions if you choose to supplement with EGCG, as products vary greatly in the amount of active ingredient. Otherwise, drink three cups of green tea daily made with one teaspoon of green tea leaves per cup of hot water. If you're not wild about the flavor, try a few different kinds. Try it iced or hot. Add some of the natural herb stevia to sweeten it if you want a sweeter drink. I wasn't crazy about green tea the first few times I tried it, but now I love it with a fresh squeeze of lemon and a few drops of stevia over ice—voilà! Check out my Green Tea Lemonade recipe on page 243.

Saffron—Research shows that an extract of the spice saffron (*Crocus sativus*) gets to the root of sweet cravings and helps eliminate them. It appears to work by regulating brain pathways in what is now referred to as the "Feed-Feedback Cycle." In one study published in *Nutrition Research* researchers found that between-meal snacking (used as a measure of cravings) was reduced by 55 percent when participants took saffron extract.[6] It is best taken in capsule or tablet. Dose varies from one product to another, so follow package directions. This herb is optional for the Fat Blast Weekend.

LICK YOUR SUGAR CRAVINGS FOR GOOD

Are sugar cravings destroying your best weight-loss efforts? Do you want your ice cream, cake, and candy too? Now you can lick those sugar cravings for good with natural foods, nutrients, and food-timing tricks. Here are easy and natural ways to send your sweet tooth packing:

Take saffron—As you learned earlier, research shows that **Crocus sativus** extract helps to regulate brain pathways involved with cravings and feelings of fullness. Supplementing with this natural form of the spice we also know as saffron can help you nix those cravings for good. See this page for more information. It is best taken in capsule or tablet. Dose varies from one product to another, so follow package directions. This herb is optional for the Fat Blast Weekend.

Supplement with chromium—Although it is an important mineral, chromium is often overlooked. It helps maintain strong arteries, blood, and heart health, and it also plays a significant role in alleviating a "sweet tooth." Chromium lessens cravings, mood swings, and weight gain linked to fluctuating blood sugar levels because it helps to keep them balanced. Chromium also plays an important role in energy production in our

continues

continued

bodies, so supplementing with chromium can give energy levels a boost too. Chromium is also naturally found in many whole grains, Romaine lettuce, onions, beans, legumes, and ripe tomatoes. Supplementing with 200 to 500 micrograms of chromium daily can help reduce cravings.

Snacking—Sugar cravings often arise from low blood sugar levels. It's the body's way of letting us know that it needs more energy to fuel our cells. But eating sugar when you have sugar cravings just creates a vicious cycle that's hard to break, causing a rapid rise in blood sugar levels that will come crashing down within an hour or two, inspiring more sugar cravings. Having a healthy snack every two to three hours stabilizes blood sugar levels, stopping sugar cravings in their tracks.

Eat protein at every meal and in every snack—Protein foods break down slowly, gradually releasing energy to the body as it needs it, keeping blood sugar levels stable. Most people assume the only protein foods are meat or poultry, but that's not the case; there are many excellent vegetarian protein foods, including lentils, chickpeas, kidney beans, pinto beans, cashews, almonds, walnuts, pecans, avocados, quinoa, and so many other delicious options.

Avoid dehydration—Our body sends us messages when it needs something. Due to most people's tendency toward food, we may misinterpret dehydration as hunger pangs. I always tell my clients to drink a large glass of pure water when they have a sweet tooth and wait thirty minutes—most of the time the cravings disappear.

Increase fiber intake—Similar to protein foods, eating fiber helps to stabilize blood sugar levels to prevent rapid spikes and drops, thereby reducing or eliminating cravings altogether.

When all else fails, eat nature's candy—When nothing but something sweet will satisfy your sugar cravings, have a piece of fresh fruit. It comes with lots of minerals, vitamins, fiber, and phytonutrients that help not only to slow the absorption of its natural sugars but also with healing and improving overall health. There are so many delicious fruits to choose from. Just keep some on hand when you have a snack attack. When it comes to weight loss, the rule of thumb for fruit is always in moderation, fresh is best, frozen is next, and minimize dried. The latter concentrates the sugars, which tend to be too high for weight loss.

THE EXERCISE

The importance of exercise for the purpose of weight loss cannot be overstated. When you are detoxifying you'll be releasing many toxins that your body will need to flush out. Exercise ensures that your lymphatic system can keep up and that your bowels are eliminating any toxins that have been stirred up. Of course, the fresh burst of oxygen into your blood also helps neutralize many microbes and makes you feel more energized too.

Metabolism-Boosting Cardio

It's important that you do some form of cardiovascular activity all three days of the Fat Blast Weekend. You'll need to do at least thirty minutes a day. If you have been inactive prior to the detox, you may wish to do cardiovascular exercise for ten minutes three times each day or fifteen minutes twice a day. Whatever you choose make sure it adds up to at least thirty minutes. Also make sure that it is sufficient to boost your heart rate without making you feel like your heart is going to jump out of your chest. It should never be so intense that you cannot carry on a discussion with someone during activity. But if your goal is fat loss, then it's equally important that the exercise be sufficiently intense to burn fat.

You can choose any form of cardiovascular exercise you prefer, including brisk walking, jogging, stair climbing, cycling, spinning, or dancing. You don't need a health club membership or expensive equipment. You don't need special training or a body-hugging outfit to get fit. All you need is some motivation and a willingness to get moving. Pick a form of activity you will actually enjoy; making exercise fun means you're more likely to do it.

If you're already doing cardio, keep up the great work.

Strength Training to Target Fatty Areas

You will also need to do strength training all three days of the Fat Blast Weekend. Muscle burns fat—it's that simple. If you want to eliminate excess fat, you need to build muscle. So during the next few days start lifting weights. You don't need to buy dumbbells or other weights. Of course, you can if you want to, but even lifting grocery bags, heavy books, or heavy canned goods (you know, the ones you won't be eating during your detox!) will do.

You'll want to target all of the major muscle groups by doing various strength training exercises. Here are the ones I recommend.

Chest presses—Using a pair of weights or some canned goods, lie on the floor, facing the ceiling. Keep your knees bent and your feet flat, as indicated in Figure 8.1. Hold the weights above your chest, keeping your arms straight but not locked at the elbow. Gradually lower the dumbbells until your upper arms touch the floor, creating a 45-degree angle with your torso. Pause briefly, and then return the dumbbells to the starting position. Repeat ten times for one set. Repeat three sets.

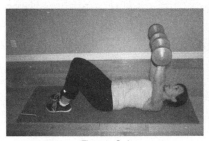

Figure 8.1

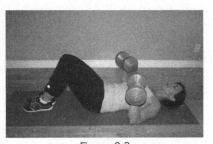

Figure 8.2

Curls—Using dumbbells or canned goods, stand in an erect position with your feet shoulder width apart, allowing the weights to hang at your sides. Now begin by bending your elbows to curl the weights up to your shoulders. Remember to keep your upper arms at your sides. Pause for a second or two, and then gradually lower the weights to the original position. Straighten your arms without locking your elbows. Complete three sets of ten repetitions. See Figure 8.3.

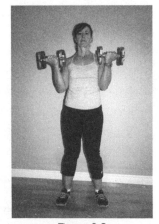

Figure 8.3

Knee lifts—Stand in an erect position with your feet shoulder width apart. Now move your arms straight out from your sides, as depicted in Figure 8.4. Lift your leg as though you are beginning to march. Your thigh should be parallel to the floor and form a 90-degree angle. Hold for a second or two, and then gradually bring your leg back into the starting position. Repeat on the other leg, completing ten repetitions on each side.

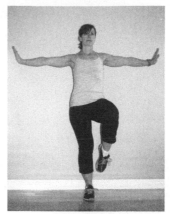

Figure 8.4

Leg lifts—Lying on the floor on your back, stretch your legs out in front of you. If you need a towel rolled up under your lower back, feel free to do so. Keep your legs in an extended position, then slowly raise them until they form an L-shape with your body. Keep your toes pointed skyward. Lower your legs slowly until they are about one inch from the floor. Pause briefly, and then lift again. Remember, do not touch your leg to the floor until you have completed this exercise ten times. Repeat on the other side. See Figures 8.5 and 8.6.

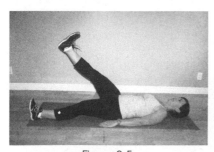

Figure 8.5

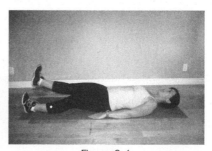

Figure 8.6

Sideways leg lifts—Lying on your left side, keeping your left elbow bent for head support and your right hand on the floor for balance, raise your right leg as high as possible. Remember, speed isn't beneficial for strength training—slower is better. Keep the rest of your body still while lifting your leg. Pause, then return the right leg to the starting position. Repeat ten times with each leg. See Figures 8.7 and 8.8.

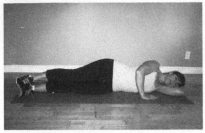

Figure 8.7

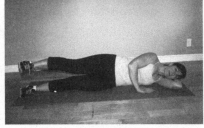

Figure 8.8

Squats—Stand in an erect position with your feet approximately shoulder width apart. Pull in your abdominal muscles while still retaining a natural arch in your lower back. Lift your arms straight out in front of you at shoulder level. Lower your body as far as you can while maintaining a seated position. Don't allow your knees to move forward farther than your toes. Pause briefly, then return to the original position. Repeat ten times. See Figures 8.9 and 8.10.

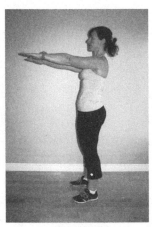

Figure 8.9

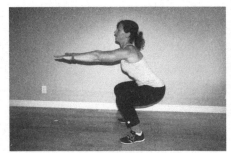

Figure 8.10

Triceps extensions—Using dumbbells or canned goods, stand in an erect
position with your feet shoulder width
apart. Keep your palms facing each other
while moving your arms over your head
until they are parallel to the floor. Hold
briefly, then straighten your arms to the
original position. Repeat ten times. See
Figure 8.11.

It's always important to be conscious
of maintaining correct posture when doing strength training. Avoid straining
your muscles by respecting your body
and its current limitations, especially

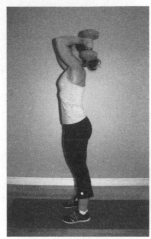

Figure 8.11

if you have any health conditions or have been sedentary. You
need to maintain the balance between surpassing your current
limitations while not doing damage to your body, particularly your
joints. If your joints are sore, it is most likely a sign to stop.

THE SPA TREATMENTS

Aromatherapy Abdominal Massage

I developed the following aromatherapy abdominal massage after
discovering a couple of exciting studies proving aromatherapy has
the power to help you lose weight.

The first study was conducted at the Department of Nursing
at the Wonkwang Health Science College in Korea. The scientists studied the effects of aromatherapy abdominal massage on
postmenopausal women. They divided the women into a group
that performed self-abdominal massage with oil, but no aromatherapy oils, and another group that performed the same self-
abdominal massage using a blend of grapefruit, lemon, and cypress
essential oils. All women performed the massage five days a week
for six weeks. The scientists found that the women who used the

essential oil blend had significantly less abdominal fat at the end of the study. Their waist measurements also dropped significantly, and they saw an improvement in their body image.

Another study from Niigata University School of Medicine in Japan showed that grapefruit and lemon essential oils activated the body's ability to burn fat and prevent further weight gain.[7]

Put the power of grapefruit, lemon, and cypress essential oils to work for you by doing the aromatherapy abdominal massage daily. Choose only high-quality essential oils (not fragrance oils, which are synthetic and offer no health benefits and may actually harm your body). Purchase grapefruit and lemon essential oils. You can add cypress, but it isn't necessary if your budget doesn't permit it or you simply can't find it. Also obtain sweet almond oil (not bitter almond oil) to use as a carrier oil for the essential oils.

Here's how to make your fat-blasting massage oil.

1. Measure two ounces of sweet almond oil in a glass measuring cup.
2. Add five drops each of pure grapefruit and lemon essential oils. Add five drops of cypress essential oil if you are using it.
3. Pour the oil blend into a glass bottle with a lid. Shake the bottle gently to blend all ingredients together.

How to perform the aromatherapy abdominal massage:

Pour a small amount of the oil blend into your hands. Rub the oil onto your abdomen in large circles, beginning just above your belly button. Massage the oil out to the left side of your belly, downward, and across the lower part of your abdomen. Then massage the oil back up the right side. Continue massaging your abdomen using firm but not forceful pressure for at least ten minutes, though you can continue longer if you'd like. See Figures 8.12 to 8.15.

Do this massage once or twice daily for all three days of the Fat Blast Weekend.

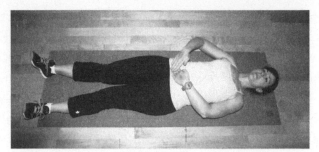

Figure 8.12

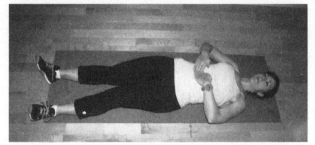

Figure 8.13

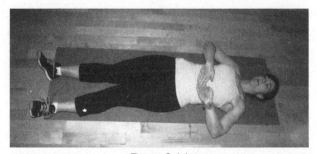

Figure 8.14

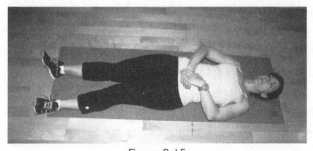

Figure 8.15

Note that many people find this massage difficult at first because it brings up emotional issues of dislike toward their bodies. But that is exactly why this massage is so valuable—it helps you reconnect to your body. To aid in this process, visualize your abdomen getting thinner. Send gratitude and love to this region of your body for all it does to keep you alive and help you every day. After all, it breaks down food and extracts nutrients to help build every cell in your body, helps you to eliminate harmful toxins that would otherwise cause serious damage, secretes life-saving enzymes and hormones to keep your body functioning properly, and so much more.

THE WEEKEND

By now you have a good understanding of foods, nutrients, herbs, exercises, and natural therapies that help with fat loss. I'll help you put together your weekend here.

Choose the foods from the list that appeal most to you. You don't need to stick to the meal plan; it is just a guideline to help you get started. I don't want this to feel arduous or for you to feel deprived. Choose a wide variety of foods for the best results and to prevent boredom on the plan.

Here's a sample of what your three-day weekend could look like.

Days one to three:

Upon rising—Drink a large glass of water (two cups) with the fresh juice of one-half lemon (optional). Add a few drops of liquid stevia if you prefer a sweeter-tasting beverage. Wait twenty minutes before eating.

Metabolism-boosting cardio

Breakfast—Some good options include the Liver Jumpstart Juice (page 242), Super-Detoxifying Green Tea Lemonade (page 243), Cranberry Green Tea Lemonade (page 243), Veggie Scramble (page 262), a soft-boiled egg with Lemon-Garlic Greens (page 252), or Chia Breakfast Tapioca (page 266).

Multivitamin

Optional nutrients

Herb (first dose of selected herbs. You can omit this step if you drink green tea at breakfast.)

Midmorning—Super-Detoxifying Green Tea Lemonade (page 243), Cranberry Green Tea Lemonade (page 243), or a cup of Love Your Liver Herbal Tea (page 244)

Snack, such as an apple, raw unsalted almonds, or celery sticks with almond butter or Herbes de Provence Cashew Cheese (page 250)

Exercise—strength training to target fatty areas

Aromatherapy abdominal massage

Lunch—Weekend Wonder Detox Signature Salad (page 258) or other large detoxifying salad. This is a good opportunity to eat more of the Top Eight Fat-Blasting Foods.

Love Your Liver Herbal Tea (page 244), the Liver Jumpstart Juice (page 242), Honey-Turmeric Tea (page 247), Ginger Chili Quinoa (page 264), or Spicy, Rice-y Detox Soup (page 260)

Optional nutrients

Herb (second dose of selected herb. You can omit this step if you drink green tea at breakfast.)

Midafternoon—Large glass of water (with lemon if desired), a cup of Super-Detoxifying Green Tea Lemonade (page 243), a cup of hot green tea, Cranberry Green Tea Lemonade (page 243), or Citrus Boost (page 241)

Snack, such as apple, raw unsalted almonds or walnuts, Cucumber-Mint Salad (page 258), an apple with almond butter, or celery sticks with almond butter or Herbes de Provence Cashew Cheese (page 250)

Dinner—Salmon Parcels (page 266) with Lemon-Garlic Greens (page 252) or Lentil Bowl (page 263) and Heirloom Tomato and Basil Salad (page 257)

Fresh cup of Celery Cucumber Juice (page 240), Liver Jumpstart Juice (page 242), or Honey-Turmeric Tea (page 247)

Herb (third dose of selected herb. You can omit this step if you drink green tea.)

After dinner—Large glass of water (with lemon if desired), a cup of Honey-Turmeric Tea (page 247), or Watermelon Ice (page 241)

Before bed—Take some quiet time to turn off the television. Find a quiet place to sit, close your eyes, and take some deep breaths.

Write in the Fat Blast Weekend Detox Journal (at the end of this chapter).

CONCLUDING THE
FAT BLAST WEEKEND

By now you've completed or are about to complete the Fat Blast Weekend. Congratulations that you are taking the time out of your busy schedule to do something healthy and healing for your body. After the Fat Blast Weekend you may wish to keep incorporating the Top Eight Fat-Burning Foods, nutrients, herbs, exercise, and spa treatment into your day-to-day life. I hope you will. Of course, you can continue to do as much or as little as you choose. Most people feel so good about the changes they've made that they keep incorporating many of them into their regular life.

You can incorporate these healthful items in whatever way works best for you. You may wish to follow the Fat Blast Weekend every weekend until you reach your weight-loss goals or to alternate weekends or even to use it as a jumping-off point to dive straight into a healthier lifestyle. If you continue, simply take a few days break from the saffron every month. And to assist you with your weight-loss goals, you may also wish to use the Love Your Liver Weekend and the Lymphomania Weekend because balancing these important bodily systems is critical for long-term health and to reach your ideal weight.

THE WORKSHEETS

The Grocery List

For easy Fat Blast Weekend prep, print this list and take it with you when you go to your local health food and grocery stores. Remember that not all of the items are essential. Purchase only the foods, nutrients, herbs, and items for the spa treatments you've selected.

Foods

Here are the fat-burning foods you'll need. Also, make sure your pantry is stocked with the essential items you learned about in Chapter 2 for any recipes you select.

— almonds
— apple cider vinegar
— avocado
— chiles
— cinnamon
— coconut (unsweetened only)
— coconut oil
— flax seeds
— flax seed oil
— grapefruit
— green tea
— legumes (beans)
— leafy greens (kale, mustard greens, spinach, spring mix, and other leafy greens)
— lemons (or lemon juice)
— olive oil (cold-pressed, extra-virgin)
— seaweed
— tomatoes
— turmeric
— walnuts
— wild salmon

Nutritional Supplements
- __ multivitamin and mineral (essential)
- __ carnitine (essential)
- __ resveratrol and isoflavones (optional; although these are two separate nutrients, they often come bottled together)
- __ grapeseed extract (optional)

Herbs Selected

Choose one or both of the following herbs:
- __ green tea
- __ saffron

Items for the Aromatherapy
Abdominal Massage Spa Treatment
- __ sweet almond oil
- __ grapefruit essential oil
- __ lemon essential oil
- __ cypress essential oil (optional)

The Fat Blast Weekend Detox Journal

You may wish to print off a copy of the journal page to make it easier to complete.

Energy: Rate your energy (from 0 to 10, with 0 meaning complete exhaustion, and 10 meaning abundant energy). Before the detox _____ After the detox _____

Pain: Rate your pain levels (from 0 to 10, with 0 meaning none, and 10 meaning unbearable, constant pain). Before the detox _____ After the detox _____

Mood: Rate your mood (from 0 to 10, with 0 meaning extremely moody, depressed, angry, or irritable, and 10 meaning extremely happy). Before the detox _____ After the detox _____

Weight: Before the detox _____ After the detox _____

Checklist of the Top Twenty Fat-Burning Foods Consumed

Try to eat at least five a day. Check the ones you ate each day.

	Day 1	Day 2	Day 3
almonds	_____	_____	_____
apple cider vinegar	_____	_____	_____
avocado	_____	_____	_____
chiles	_____	_____	_____
cinnamon	_____	_____	_____
coconut (unsweetened only)	_____	_____	_____
coconut oil	_____	_____	_____
flax seeds	_____	_____	_____
flax seed oil	_____	_____	_____
grapefruit	_____	_____	_____
green tea	_____	_____	_____
legumes (beans)	_____	_____	_____
leafy greens (kale, mustard greens, spinach, spring mix, and other leafy greens)	_____	_____	_____
lemons (or lemon juice)	_____	_____	_____
olive oil (cold-pressed, extra-virgin)	_____	_____	_____
seaweed	_____	_____	_____
tomatoes	_____	_____	_____
turmeric	_____	_____	_____
walnuts	_____	_____	_____
wild salmon	_____	_____	_____

Selected Nutrients

Be sure to take the multivitamin and carnitine each day. Write down any additional nutrients you've opted to take throughout the detox. Remember, you don't need to take all of them. Check off each day you take them.

	Day 1	Day 2	Day 3
multivitamin and mineral	_____	_____	_____
carnitine	_____	_____	_____
resveratrol and isoflavones (optional)	_____	_____	_____
grapeseed extract (optional)	_____	_____	_____

Selected Herbs

Indicate the one to two herbs you've selected to take throughout the detox. Check off each day you take them. Most herbs need to be taken three times daily.

	Day 1	Day 2	Day 3
green tea	_____	_____	_____
saffron	_____	_____	_____

Exercise

Check off each time you complete cardiovascular and weight workouts. Make sure to do it every day.

	Day 1	Day 2	Day 3
cardiovascular (thirty minutes or more)	_____	_____	_____
weights	_____	_____	_____

Selected Spa Treatment(s)

Check off each time you complete the fat-burning spa treatment. It's not necessary to it, but, if you do, make sure you do it every day.

	Day 1	Day 2	Day 3
aromatherapy abdominal massage	_____	_____	_____

Observations and Thoughts

Day 1: _____

_____

_____

_____

Day 2: _____

_____

_____

_____

Day 3: _____

_____

_____

_____

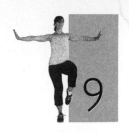

KEEPING THE DETOX SPIRIT ALIVE AFTER THE WEEKEND'S OVER

Learning to respect and care for your body is a major step toward healing. Your body is not just a piece of machinery in which components can be cut out or other components added; rather, every part of your body works together with an intelligence that is both mind-boggling and miraculous.

In a single second your body coordinates billions of simultaneous processes that control every chemical, energetic, electric, and mechanical process to keep you alive. Trillions of cells work at lightning speed to overcome infection, mend broken bones, and heal wounds. Healthy cells replenish dying or dysfunctional cells every second to create a healthier body. Your skin is totally renewed every twenty-eight days. You literally have a new heart every thirty days. Your lungs regenerate every seventy days.

When you eliminate toxins from your cells, tissues, organs, and organ systems you will experience a cleaner and clearer you. Your energy will soar, pain will lessen or disappear, your mind will be clearer, you'll sleep better, and your movement will be freer. Even your moods will improve. Your skin will clear, and fine wrinkles may recede. Your body will feel lighter, and this lightness will expand outward into your outlook on life. It seems impossible that detoxification can do so many things, but remember what detoxification ultimately is: taking time out from the hectic pace of life to take care of your body, to say "my body is worth treating well." And this attitude as well as better-functioning, cleaner cells combine to create a stronger, healthier, happier you. It allows you to discover and fulfill the potential that is *you*.

We are not deficient in pharmaceutical drugs. We do not have deficiencies of aspirin, warfarin, or other chemicals. Our symptoms are signs that our bodies need more attention, more nutrients, fewer toxins, pure water, deeper breathing, and more movement. We are complex physical, emotional, intellectual, energetic, and spiritual beings. Our bodies have developed sophisticated detoxification mechanisms, but in our industrial age they can use a boost to function at optimal levels throughout our life.

Although improvements and even transformations may occur in a single weekend, the reality is that our bodies may need more than that to counterbalance the years of toxins, unhealthy eating habits, and a sedentary lifestyle. You can detox one weekend out of every month or once in a season, or you can detox every weekend if you want. The choice is yours. You can stick with one specific detox until you see your symptoms in the quiz in Chapter 2 reduce, or you can try different ones to give all your organs a boost.

There's no limit to the amount you can detoxify your body provided you give it the healthy fuel it needs to maintain and achieve health. Of course, there are times in life when you'll need to take a break from detoxification. These times include pregnancy, breastfeeding, if you're suffering from an eating disorder, or if you have a serious illness like diabetes. Other than that, you can periodically retake the quiz in Chapter 2 to guide you on the next path of your healing journey to restore your health one weekend at a time.

The sixteenth-century German-Swiss physician and founder of toxicology, Paracelsus, said, "The art of healing comes from nature, not from the physician." Although hundreds of years have passed and we live in a world increasingly separated from nature and our own true nature, these words were never truer. Remove the barriers to health (toxins) and refuel every cell in your body with fresh, wholesome foods, and you will restore great health. Love your body, and it will love you back.

Wishing you great health and happiness,
Michelle Schoffro Cook

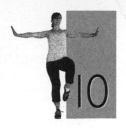

RECIPES

You'll find lots of delicious detoxifying recipes for all of the Weekend Wonder Detoxes here. Most recipes don't require any special equipment, although you'll need a juicer for the juice recipes. There are many excellent affordable juicers under $50. And it's a frequent item at garage sales if that price is too steep for your budget.

Some recipes call for "green powder." There are many varieties available. Be sure to choose one that is free of sweeteners, fillers, and gluten. If it doesn't say "gluten-free" on the label, it probably isn't. Some of my preferred choices include chlorella powder or spirulina powder.

I'd like to thank my good friend Cobi Slater, PhD, DNM, RHT, ROHP, RNCP, a board-certified doctor of natural medicine, at drcobi.com, for sharing some of her delicious, nutritious, and detoxifying recipes.

BEVERAGES

I encourage you to choose organic fruits and vegetables for the juices. Not only are they better for you, but you'll also save yourself the time peeling them. Most of the nutrients are near the skin's surface, so it's better to wash and forgo peeling. Cut the produce into sizes suitable for your specific juicer. Some require one- to two-inch chunks or slices, whereas others don't need any chopping at all. Check your owner's manual if you're not sure.

Cucumber Mint Refresh

This supercleansing recipe is perfect on a hot day.

• SERVES 1 •

1 large cucumber
½ apple (optional)
Sprig fresh mint

Blend all ingredients in a blender with some water or push through a juicer. Serve over ice. Drink immediately.

Carrot Celery Juice

This detoxifying juice contains lots of skin-purifying beta carotene and anti-inflammatory celery.

• SERVES 1 •

4 to 5 large carrots
2 stalks celery
½ apple (optional)

Push all ingredients through a juicer. Drink immediately.

Celery Cucumber Juice

Celery Cucumber Juice is a super-anti-inflammatory cocktail that helps every detox organ.

• SERVES 1 •

4 stalks celery
1 cucumber
½ apple

Push all ingredients through a juicer. Drink immediately.

Watermelon Ice

Watermelon contains detoxifying glutathione, which helps neutralize toxins. It is also a good source of the anticancer compound lycopene.

• SERVES 2 •

4 cups seedless watermelon, skin removed, chopped into chunks
6 ice cubes (more if desired)
Sprig fresh mint (optional)

Blend all ingredients in a blender. Serve over ice. Drink immediately.

Cantaloupe Ice

Packed with skin-enriching and immune-boosting beta carotene, cantaloupe is as refreshing as it is detoxifying.

• SERVES 2 •

4 cups cantaloupe, seeded and skin removed, chopped into chunks
6 ice cubes (more if desired)

Blend all ingredients in a blender. Serve over ice. Drink immediately.

Citrus Boost

This juice helps detoxify your blood, liver, kidneys, lymphatic system, and intestines. It can be made with a fruit and vegetable juicer, a citrus juicer, a high-powered blender, or just a citrus reamer, whichever you prefer.

• SERVES 1 •

1 grapefruit
½ lemon

I cup water

A few drops of liquid stevia to sweeten (optional)

In a juicer or high-powered blender, juice the grapefruit and lemon, and add the water. Sweeten with stevia to taste, if desired. Pour over ice, and drink immediately. If you're using a blender or traditional juicer, you'll need to peel the fruit. If you're using a special citrus juicer, you can leave the peel on.

Liver Jumpstart Juice

This juice is aptly named because it really helps with liver detoxification. But the vitamin- and mineral-rich greens are also great for any of the detoxes.

• SERVES I •

Handful fresh dandelion greens

Handful fresh lettuce greens

I beet

2 carrots

I cucumber

I small apple

Push all ingredients through a juicer. Drink immediately.

Cranberry Pear Juice

The lymphatic system and kidneys really benefit from the cranberries in this juice. The pear sweetens it slightly.

• SERVES I •

I cup fresh or frozen cranberries

I pear, cored

I cup water

Blend all ingredients in a blender until smooth. Drink immediately. Add a few drops of stevia to sweeten, if desired.

Super-Detoxifying Green Tea Lemonade

Not sure you can skip your morning coffee while detoxifying? Try this green tea lemonade. I created this recipe because green tea is a serious superfood, and I really couldn't stand the taste of it. I love this delicious drink, though. Every green tea hater I've given it to thinks it's great. It is sweetened with the herb stevia to make it naturally sweet without affecting blood sugar levels. If you're trying to lose weight, it has lots of fat-busting properties to make it the ideal weight-loss beverage.

• SERVES 2 TO 4 •

1 quart or liter water
6 green tea bags
4 lemons, juiced
10 drops liquid stevia (or to taste)
Ice

Bring the water to boil. Add the tea bags, and let them steep for about 5 to 10 minutes. While the tea is steeping, mix the lemon juice with the stevia. Add ice to the tea, and allow it to cool before adding the lemon juice–stevia mixture. Stir until mixed, and enjoy served over ice.

Cranberry Green Tea Lemonade

This is a variation on the Super-Detoxifying Green Tea Lemonade. The addition of cranberries helps to further strengthen the kidneys and lymphatic system.

• SERVES 2 TO 4 •

1 quart or liter water
6 green tea bags
4 lemons, juiced
10 drops liquid stevia (or to taste)
Ice
1 cup fresh or frozen cranberries

Bring the water to boil. Add the tea bags, and let them steep for about 5 to 10 minutes. While the tea is steeping, mix the lemon juice with the stevia. Add ice to the tea, and allow it to cool before adding the lemon juice–stevia mixture. Pour into a blender with the cranberries. Blend and serve.

Mom's Energy Smoothie

Here is one of my mom's excellent recipes, which she uses to boost her energy. It's packed with energy-giving vitamins and minerals, plant nutrients, and fiber, all of which can help you get going in the morning or midday when you need a boost. Don't be alarmed by the less-than-appetizing color—this smoothie tastes great. Skip the banana if you're trying to lose weight.

• SERVES 2 •

1 banana
1 tablespoon ground flax seeds
1 tablespoon green powder (such as spirulina, chlorella, or green juice
     powder) or 1 cup of fresh leafy greens
1 teaspoon coconut oil or flax seed oil
1½ cups frozen fruit (blueberries, strawberries, mangoes,
     or purple grapes)
2 cups water (use more or less water, depending on preferred
     consistency)

Place all ingredients in a blender, and blend until smooth. Drink immediately.

Love Your Liver Herbal Tea

This herbal tea gives your liver a serious boost. You can use it in place of taking herbal capsules, tablets, or tinctures that are recommended for the Love Your Liver Weekend.

• SERVES 3 •

1 teaspoon dried dandelion root

1 teaspoon dried Oregon grape root

1 teaspoon dried mint

4 cups water

Mix together all ingredients in a medium saucepan, and bring to a boil. Reduce the heat, and let it simmer, covered, for 15 minutes. Strain and serve. Drink 1 cup 3 times daily for best results. Sweeten with a few drops of stevia, if desired.

Note: These herbs are available at most health food stores.

Lymphomania Herbal Tea

This herbal tea improves the flow of the lymphatic system. You can use it in place of taking herbal capsules, tablets, or tinctures that are recommended for the Lymphomania Weekend.

• SERVES 3 •

1 teaspoon dried echinacea

1 teaspoon dried astragalus

1 teaspoon dried cleavers

1 teaspoon dried mint

4 cups water

Mix together all ingredients in a medium saucepan, and bring to a boil. Reduce the heat, and let it simmer, covered, for 15 minutes. Strain and serve. Drink 1 cup 3 times daily for best results. Sweeten with a few drops of stevia, if desired.

Note: These herbs are available at most health food stores.

Kidney Herbal Tea

This herbal tea cleanses the kidneys while nourishing them with critical nutrients. You can use it in place of taking herbal capsules, tablets, or tinctures that are recommended for the Kidney Flush Weekend.

• SERVES 3 •

1 teaspoon dried bearberry
1 teaspoon dried buchu
1 teaspoon dried cleavers
1 teaspoon dried dandelion
1 teaspoon dried mint
4 cups water

Mix together all ingredients in a medium saucepan, and bring to a boil. Reduce the heat, and let it simmer, covered, for 15 minutes. Strain and serve. Drink 1 cup 3 times daily for best results. Sweeten with a few drops of stevia, if desired.

These herbs are available at most health food stores.

Colon Cleanse Herbal Tea

This herbal tea stimulates the intestines to eliminate toxins while also killing any harmful microbes that may live there. You can use it in place of taking herbal capsules, tablets, or tinctures that are recommended for the Colon Cleanse Weekend.

• SERVES 3 •

1 teaspoon dried cascara sagrada
1 teaspoon dried licorice root
1 teaspoon dried white walnut
4 cups water

Mix together all ingredients in a medium saucepan, and bring to a boil. Reduce the heat, and let it simmer, covered, for 15 minutes. Strain and serve. Drink 1 cup 3 times daily for best results. Sweeten with a few drops of stevia, if desired.

These herbs are available at most health food stores.

Skin Rejuvenation Herbal Tea

This herbal tea is supercleansing for the skin. You can use it in place of taking herbal capsules, tablets, or tinctures that are recommended for the Skin Rejuvenation Weekend.

• SERVES 3 •

1 teaspoon dried yellow dock
1 teaspoon dried cleavers
1 teaspoon dried mint
4 cups water

Mix together all ingredients in a medium saucepan, and bring to a boil. Reduce the heat, and let it simmer, covered, for 15 minutes. Strain and serve. Drink 1 cup 3 times daily for best results. Sweeten with a few drops of stevia, if desired.

These herbs are available at most health food stores.

Honey-Turmeric Tea

Turmeric is healing to every organ and organ system in the body largely due to its anti-inflammatory component called cucumin.

Honey
Turmeric (available in most health food stores)

In a food processor, mix equal parts honey and turmeric until blended. Store in a jar with a lid. Use one heaping teaspoon of the mixture in a cup of hot water to drink as tea. Stir occasionally to prevent the turmeric from settling on the bottom.

APPETIZERS, DIPS, AND SPREADS

Dairy-Free Yogurt

Many people find that fermented soy, like this dairy-free yogurt, is much easier to tolerate than nonfermented products. Making your own dairy-free yogurt is easier than you think. You don't need any expensive equipment or yogurt makers, either. Just use a 1½-quart ceramic crock or bowl (metal interferes with the natural culturing process). You'll also need a high-quality dairy-free probiotic powder, which is available from most health food stores and many online stores.

The process works well with organic soy milk or coconut milk—both are delicious. Don't use soy unless it's certified organic, as most soy is genetically modified. Rice milk and almond milk are too thin. If you use canned coconut milk, be sure to mix it thoroughly first to blend the coconut water and the milk together. When canned coconut milk cultures, the yogurt rises to the top while the liquid drops below, making it a bit tricky to separate, but not impossible.

1 quart or liter organic soy milk or coconut milk
1 teaspoon probiotic powder

Heat the soy milk to lukewarm or body temperature, but not too hot, or else the yogurt cultures will be destroyed. Pour into a clean ceramic crock or bowl.

Add the probiotic powder, and stir until dissolved. Cover and set in a warm area for 6 to 10 hours, depending on the temperature and your preference for thicker or thinner yogurt or the level of tartness you prefer. Longer times and warmer temperatures will produce thicker yogurt and increase the tartness; however, do not heat the milk or probiotics, as heat will kill the bacteria.

Carefully remove the lid. Due to the proliferation of probiotics, the "milk" should have separated into a thick yogurt and a thin liquid. Pour off the thin liquid or scoop out the thick yogurt, depending on whether the thin liquid floats or drops to the bottom.

Enjoy the many health-rejuvenating properties of probiotics without the dairy, excessive amounts of sugar, and higher price tag of commercial yogurt (most of which don't actually contain live cultures). Dairy-free yogurt is excellent with berries, peaches, sprinkled with raw walnuts and drizzled with honey, in a smoothie, or with lemon juice and a little grated onion and cucumber (tzatziki). The yogurt will store in a sealed container in the fridge for about 1 week.

Sweet Potato Fries

This alternative to French fries tastes better and is far better for you than the original. You can use either yams or sweet potatoes. If you can't tell them apart, yams are a creamy yellow on the inside, whereas sweet potatoes are a bright salmon-orange color inside. Sweet potatoes are high in beta carotene, vitamins C and B6, as well as potassium, iron, and magnesium. Their rich orange color is the easy way to know that they are high in beta carotene, the precursor to vitamin A.

• SERVES 2 TO 4 •

4 yams or sweet potatoes, scrubbed and unpeeled
2 tablespoons extra-virgin olive oil
1 teaspoon unrefined sea salt

Preheat oven to 300°. Line a baking sheet with unbleached parchment paper or lightly grease with extra-virgin olive oil or coconut oil.

Cut yams into strips similar to French fries. Try to cut them uniformly so they'll cook evenly. Place in a large bowl, drizzle with the olive oil, and sprinkle with salt. Toss until evenly coated.

Place the fries in a single layer on a prepared baking sheet, and bake at 300° for 30 minutes. Turn them over, and bake for another 30 minutes or until lightly browned.

Better Than Butter

This Better Than Butter has all of the health benefits of medium-chain tri-glycerides in coconut oil (fat-burning, thyroid-balancing, and infection-killing) and all the benefits of flax seed oil (liver boosting, lymph cleansing, and anti-inflammatory). Serve this soft, healthier butter substitute on warm bread or on steamed or roasted vegetables after they're cooked. It's simple to make and stores well in the fridge.

• MAKES ABOUT 1 CUP •

½ cup organic extra-virgin coconut oil ·
½ cup organic cold-pressed flax seed oil

In a small saucepan, over low heat, liquefy the coconut oil. Immediately remove from the heat, and add the flax seed oil, stirring until well mixed.
Pour into a serving container (preferably glass), and refrigerate until firm.

MAKE AHEAD: Store in an airtight container in the refrigerator for up to 6 months.

VARIATION: Stir in a handful of chopped fresh basil, minced garlic, or chopped cilantro immediately after adding the flax seed oil for a flavorful "butter."

Herbes de Provence Cashew Cheese

This cheese is so delicious that no one will know it's a healthy, dairy-free option. It is an excellent dish to serve at parties and family gatherings. This recipe offers all the benefits of yogurt and helps to balance your bowel flora. Although it requires time for fermentation, it only takes about 5 to 10 minutes of preparation time. Probiotic powder is available in most health food stores and is sometimes called L. acidophilus or flora.

• MAKES APPROXIMATELY 2 CUPS •

2 cups raw, unsalted cashews, soaked overnight, about 10 to 12 hours
1 teaspoon probiotics powder or 2 capsules probiotics, opened and
    dissolved in 1 cup pure water
1 teaspoon Celtic sea salt or Himalayan crystal salt (or more to taste,
    if desired)
1 to 2 teaspoons onion powder
¼ teaspoon ground nutmeg
2 to 3 teaspoons herbes de Provence seasoning blend

In a blender or food processor, blend the soaked cashews with the probiotic powder and water mixture. Place in a glass bowl, covered with a clean cloth, and let rest for 10 to 14 hours to ferment.

Stir in the salt, onion powder, and nutmeg until well mixed. Form the cheese into a ball or press in a springform pan. Roll into the herbes de Provence to coat or press the herb mixture onto the cheese. Serve with vegetable crudité.

Chickpea Bread

This is a delicious gluten-free, dairy-free, high-fiber, high-protein bread that is delicious served warm with Better Than Butter or Herbes de Provence Cashew Cheese. It is an excellent cleanser for the intestines, which means it also helps cleanse the blood.

• SERVES 10 TO 12 •

3 cups chickpea flour
1 cup tapioca flour
1½ teaspoons baking soda
¼ cup coconut sap (coconut sugar)
⅓ cup olive oil, plus more for greasing pan if not
    using parchment paper
1 cup almond milk
3 eggs
Dash unrefined sea salt

Preheat oven to 350°. Line a standard 9 x 4-inch bread pan with unbleached parchment paper or in a pan greased with coconut oil or olive oil. Mix all ingredients in a food processor until smooth. Pour into the pan, and bake at 350° for 35 minutes, or until a toothpick comes out clean.

It lasts about 3 days, longer if refrigerated.

Chili Lime Green Beans

These sweet and spicy green beans are sure to please even green bean haters. It is one of my favorite vegetable recipes.

• SERVES 1 TO 2 •

1 tablespoon extra-virgin olive oil
1 to 2 handfuls fresh green or yellow beans, chopped into 1-inch pieces
    (about 2 cups chopped)
1 small fresh cayenne chili, minced
1 small fresh garlic clove
Pinch unrefined sea salt
1 teaspoon honey
½ lime

Place first 6 ingredients in a medium saucepan. Sauté together over low to medium heat until beans are al dente, about 15 minutes. Remove from the heat, and squeeze the lime juice over the beans. Serve immediately.

Lemon-Garlic Greens

If you're not a fan of greens, try this recipe before you write them off altogether. Even greens haters love this recipe. It's quick and easy and an excellent way to get more detox superfoods into your diet.

• SERVES 2 •

1 tablespoon extra-virgin olive oil

1 large bunch kale or chard, washed and coarsely chopped
   (if using kale, remove stems and use leafy parts only. You can
   save the stems for a juice.)
1 garlic clove, minced
2 tablespoons fresh lemon juice
Pinch or two unrefined sea salt

Heat the oil on medium in a large skillet with a lid, being careful not to allow it to smoke. Add the greens to the skillet with a small amount of water. Cover and cook 3 minutes, or until the greens have turned a bright green color and softened. Add the garlic, stirring frequently, for 1 to 2 more minutes. Remove from the heat, and toss the greens with the lemon juice and sea salt. Serve immediately.

Portobello Mushroom Gravy

We don't typically think of gravy as healthy or suitable for cleansing, but this one is! I love the rich, savory flavor of rosemary and Portobello mushroom. And forget what you've heard about homemade gravy being difficult to make—it's a cinch. It's amazing served over Roasted Red Pepper Chickpea Mash.

• MAKES 2 CUPS •

3 tablespoons extra-virgin olive oil, divided
1 small onion, finely minced
1 Portobello mushroom, washed, stem removed, and finely chopped
1 sprig fresh rosemary
1 sprig fresh thyme (optional)
2 tablespoons gluten-free flour
2 cups water
Unrefined sea salt

In a small pot over low-medium heat, sauté 1 tablespoon of olive oil, the onions, mushrooms, and sprigs of rosemary and thyme, if desired. Sauté until the onions are lightly browned and the mushrooms are soft, about 15 minutes. Remove the rosemary and thyme sprigs. Add the remaining oil and flour. Mix together until there are no flour lumps. Slowly add the water, whisking constantly until thickened without any flour lumps. Add salt to taste.

It will last in the refrigerator covered for about a week.

SALADS AND SOUPS

Create Health-Building Gourmet Salads in Minutes

If you avoid salads at any cost, thinking they consist only of iceberg lettuce and a couple of slices of starchy tomato topped with some chemical and sugar-laden bottled dressing, you will be happy to learn that with minimal effort you can create salads that inspire health AND your taste buds.

These excellent salads can be gourmet meals in themselves. I compiled the following list of possible salad ingredients to prevent boredom. It is just the beginning. The idea is to be creative. This list is just to help you get started.

Salad bases (Choose one or more—for 2 servings, 2 to 4 generous cups of vegetables or greens is a good baseline or 1 cup for grains, but obviously you can tailor to your own appetite)

beetroot (grated)	radicchio
Boston lettuce	Romaine lettuce
brown rice (cooked)	seaweed (such as arame,
endive	nori, or wakami)
grated cabbage	sprouts (such as alfalfa,
leaf lettuce	mung bean, or red clover)
mixed greens	watercress
quinoa (cooked)	wild rice

Mix-ins (pick three or more—for 2 servings, 1 cup of vegetables or ½ cup of fruit is a good baseline, but, again, you can tailor to your own appetite)

alfalfa sprouts
apples (sliced or grated)
avocado
bell peppers (red, green, or
    yellow)
blackberries
blueberries
broccoli (finely chopped)
broccoli sprouts
carrots (julienned, roasted,
    or grated)
celery
celery root
chickpeas
cucumber slices
edible flowers (e.g.,
    nasturtiums, violas, or
    pansies)
fenugreek sprouts
grapefruit slices
great northern beans

kidney beans
lima beans
mung bean sprouts
mushrooms (raw or cooked)
olives
onion (minced)
onion sprouts
orange slices
pea shoots
peas (fresh)
pinto beans
pomegranate seeds
radishes
raspberries
red clover sprouts
scallions
strawberries
sweet potato (grated or
    roasted)
tomatoes
zucchini (grated or roasted)

Toppings (pick one or more—for 2 servings, use a handful of nuts, seed, or grated veggies or about 1 tablespoon freshly chopped herbs)

almond slices
carrots (grated)
fresh basil (chopped)
fresh cilantro (chopped)
fresh mint (chopped)
fresh parsley (chopped)
hazelnuts (chopped)

herbs (such as thyme,
    oregano, or minced garlic)
pine nuts
pumpkin seeds
sesame seeds
sunflower seeds

Dressings (pick one—for 2 servings, use 2 to 4 tablespoons dressing)

balsamic vinegar

oil and lemon juice

olive oil

Your favorite homemade dressing (see suggestions below or check out my website, drmichellecook .com, for more options)

Ways to Turn Your Salad into a Fat-Blasting Salad

1. Add 1 or more of the Top Twenty Fat-Burning Foods, which include:

almonds

apple cider vinegar

avocado

chiles

cinnamon

coconut (unsweetened only)

coconut oil

flax seeds

flax seed oil

grapefruit

green tea (can be used as a tofu marinade or an ingredient in dressings)

legumes (beans)

leafy greens (kale, mustard greens, spinach, spring mix, and other leafy greens)

lemons (or lemon juice)

olive oil (cold-pressed, extra-virgin)

seaweed

tomatoes

turmeric

walnuts

wild salmon

2. Add at least one protein-rich topping (about 6 ounces, or the size of a deck of cards), which include:

almond slices or presoaked raw almonds

anchovies

black beans

Brazil nuts (raw, unsalted)

cashews (raw, unsalted)

chicken (organic only)

chickpeas

edamame (organic only)

eggs (hard- or soft-boiled, organic only)

flax seeds (ground)

great northern beans

hempseeds (ground)

kidney beans

lentils

lima beans

macadamia nuts
    (raw, unsalted)

mung bean sprouts

navy beans

pecans (raw, unsalted)

pinto beans

pistachios (raw, unsalted)

pumpkin seeds

quinoa (cooked)

Romano beans

sesame seeds

sunflower seeds
    (raw, unsalted)

tempeh (organic only)

tofu (organic only)

turkey breast
    (organic only)

walnuts (raw, unsalted)

wild salmon

3. Dress your salad. Avoid bottled dressings altogether, as most are full of junk ingredients that should never be consumed. Make your own by using 2 to 3 parts cold-pressed oil with 1 part acid-like lemon juice, lime juice, or apple cider vinegar. Making your own dressings is much easier than you think. Use a glass jar, add 1 part of the acid you selected and 2 or 3 parts of the oil, depending on preference. Cover with a lid, and shake until mixed. Or blend with a small hand blender. You can also add a handful of berries or fresh or dried herbs for a burst of flavor and fat-burning capabilities. Try some of the salad dressing recipes on page 259. Flax seed oil is a particularly good fat-burning oil choice.

Heirloom Tomato and Basil Salad

When tomatoes are in season this is my go-to recipe to enjoy them. The combination of flavors is better than any of the individual ingredients. My husband didn't like tomatoes until he tried this recipe, and now he eats this salad regularly.

• SERVES 2 •

5 medium to large heirloom tomatoes (or equivalent in small
    heirloom tomatoes)
1 garlic clove

Handful fresh basil
1 tablespoon extra-virgin olive oil
1 teaspoon unrefined sea salt

Coarsely chop the tomatoes and place in a medium bowl. Mince the garlic and basil, and add to the heirloom tomatoes. Top with olive oil and sea salt. Mix together, and let stand for about 5 minutes to allow flavors to mingle. Serve.

Cucumber-Mint Salad

This is a refreshing alternative to lettuce salads and a perfect choice for a hot summer day.

• SERVES 2 TO 4 •

2 large cucumbers
Handful fresh mint
1 tablespoon olive oil
½ lime, juiced
½ teaspoon unrefined sea salt

Chop the cucumbers into 1-inch chunks and place in a medium bowl. Mince the mint, and add to the cucumbers. Add the remaining ingredients. Mix together, and let stand for about 5 minutes to allow the flavors to mingle. Serve.

Weekend Wonder Detox Signature Salad

If you're looking for a superdetoxifying and supertasting salad to enjoy throughout your weekend detox, this one is sure to please. It is packed with nutrients for every detoxification system. But you might forget how detoxifying it is when you taste how delicious it is.

• SERVES 1 TO 2 •

Dressing

¼ cup cold-pressed flax seed oil
½ cup extra-virgin olive oil
⅓ cup freshly squeezed lemon juice
Pinch unrefined sea salt
Handful fresh cilantro
Handful fresh parsley
1 garlic clove
1 teaspoon honey

Salad

2 cups leafy greens, your choice
½ carrot, grated
1 small beet, grated
Handful raw, unsalted pumpkin seeds

Blend all dressing ingredients together in a blender.

Assemble the leafy greens, grated carrot, and beet on a large plate or bowl. Top with a small amount of dressing and pumpkin seeds.

Salade du Provence Dressing

This dressing is versatile and is a classic dressing that tends to go with just about anything.

• SERVES 4 TO 6 •

¼ cup balsamic vinegar
¾ cup extra-virgin olive oil
1 teaspoon honey
1 teaspoon mustard
1 teaspoon herbes de Provence (available in most health food stores)
Dash unrefined sea salt
Dash freshly ground black pepper

Mix all ingredients together in a jar and shake, or blend together in a blender.

Lasts about 2 weeks stored in the refrigerator.

Citrus Power Dressing

I'm not a huge fan of oranges, but somehow they work beautifully in this recipe. The flavors are dynamic and great on greens. The sweet and tart flavors tend to go well with most foods.

• SERVES 8 TO 10 •

Juice of ½ grapefruit
Juice of ½ lemon or lime
Juice of 1 orange
½ cup extra-virgin olive oil
Dash unrefined sea salt
Dash freshly ground black pepper

Mix all ingredients together in a jar and shake, or blend together in a blender.

Lasts about 2 weeks stored in the refrigerator.

Spicy, Rice-y Detox Soup

Even if you're not a fan of brown rice, you'll love this soup. It is rich, hearty, and supercleansing. The rosemary and garlic boost your liver, while the celery and jalapeños alleviate inflammation and help keep your lymphatic system moving.

• SERVES 4 TO 6 •

2 tablespoons olive oil
1 large or 2 medium onions, chopped
2 stalks celery, chopped

2 carrots, chopped

2 sprigs rosemary

2 garlic cloves, minced

½ jalapeño, minced

½ cup brown rice

9 cups water

1 teaspoon sea salt

In a large pot over low to medium heat sauté the olive oil, onions, celery, and carrots until soft, about 10 to 14 minutes. Add all remaining ingredients. Cover and bring to a boil, about 5 to 10 minutes. Reduce the heat, and simmer until the rice is cooked, about 45 minutes. Serve.

You can freeze this soup for a quick and easy meal in a pinch. It lasts about 4 days in the fridge.

Thai Coconut Vegetable Soup

Courtesy of Dr. Cobi Slater, this recipe is a detoxifying take on a Thai classic.

• SERVES 2 •

2 cups vegetable or chicken stock

1 14-ounce can coconut milk

1 teaspoon crushed red chili flakes

6 to 8 garlic cloves, crushed

1 small onion, cut into half moons

1 red bell pepper, cut into strips

1 medium zucchini, cut in half lengthwise, then sliced

2 cups thinly sliced bok choy leaves or cabbage leaves

½ cup chopped cilantro

Sea salt or Herbamare, to taste

Place the stock into a 4-quart pot over medium heat. Add the coconut milk, red chili flakes, garlic, onion, and bell pepper. Simmer for 15 minutes, covered, or until the vegetables are just tender.

Add the zucchini, and simmer 5 minutes more. Remove the pot from the heat, and add the sliced bok choy leaves, cilantro, and salt. Garnish with extra red chili flakes, if desired.

Stores about 4 days in the fridge. Freezes well.

ENTRÉES

Veggie Scramble

Think you can't stand tofu? This veggie scramble is a delicious alternative to scrambled eggs with veggies added. It's great for breakfast or as a quick and easy dinner.

• SERVES 2 •

8 ounces firm organic tofu, crumbled

1 ½ teaspoons ground turmeric

1 teaspoon unrefined sea salt

½ teaspoon ground cumin (optional)

5 tomatoes, quartered

2 tablespoons extra-virgin olive oil

1 large onion, chopped

1 small sweet potato, chopped (optional)

2 celery stalks, chopped

1 red bell pepper, chopped

1 green bell pepper, chopped

Combine the tofu, turmeric, salt, and cumin, if desired, in a bowl; set aside. In a blender or food processor, purée the tomatoes; set aside.

Heat the oil over medium-low heat in a large skillet, making sure it never smokes. Sauté the onions until softened, about 5 to 10 minutes. Add the sweet potato, if desired, and sauté until tender, about 15 minutes. Add the celery and bell peppers; sauté until tender, about 2 to 4 minutes. Add the seasoned tofu, and sauté until heated through, about 1 minute. Stir in the tomato purée, cover, and cook for 5 to 10 minutes or until the purée is heated through and the flavors have blended.

Serve on its own for breakfast or as a delicious and quick dinner.

Roasted Red Pepper Chickpea Mash

Mashed potatoes tend to cause weight gain. The acrylamides that form in white potatoes while cooking them are anything but healthy. I developed this recipe as a high-protein, high-fiber alternative to mashed potatoes. The roasted red pepper adds amazing flavor and extra vitamin C. Serve with Portobello Mushroom Gravy for a delicious treat.

• SERVES 2 TO 4 •

2 tablespoons extra-virgin olive oil
1 medium onion, chopped
1 red bell pepper, chopped
1 sprig rosemary
2 19-ounce cans chickpeas, drained and rinsed
1 cup water
1 teaspoon unrefined sea salt

Heat the oil and sauté the onion, bell pepper, and rosemary in a large pot over low to medium heat until the onion is lightly browned, around 15 minutes. Place the chickpeas, water, salt, and sautéed onion–red pepper mixture in a food processor, and purée until smooth. Return to the pot to heat, adding a small amount of water if necessary to prevent sticking.

Serve with Portobello Mushroom Gravy for a delicious, detoxifying alternative to mashed potatoes and gravy.

Lentil Bowl

Don't underestimate how good these simple ingredients can be when combined. It's a snap to make and a superdetoxifying recipe to enjoy on the Weekend Wonder Detox.

• SERVES 2 TO 4 •

2 tablespoons extra-virgin olive oil
2 medium or 3 small onions, chopped
3 cups cooked lentils, drained
1 garlic clove, minced
1 teaspoon unrefined sea salt

Heat the oil over medium-low heat in a large skillet, making sure it never smokes. Add the onions, and sauté until lightly browned, about 10 to 15 minutes. Place in a medium bowl, and add the lentils, garlic, and salt; mix well. Serve warm.

Ginger Chili Quinoa

I was tired of quinoa recipes that all tasted alike, so I developed this Asian-inspired recipe, and now it's my favorite way to eat this superfood. It's packed with flavor and anti-inflammatory ginger and cayenne, making it the perfect detox dinner.

• SERVES 2 TO 4 •

1 cup quinoa, rinsed
1¾ cups water
1 small garlic clove, minced
1 small fresh cayenne chili, minced
½ teaspoon unrefined sea salt
1-inch piece ginger, peeled and minced
1 small onion, chopped
1 tablespoon coconut oil

Mix all the ingredients in a small saucepan. Cover, place on medium-high heat, and bring to a boil. Stir, cover, and reduce the heat to a minimum; allow to simmer for 20 minutes or until the water is absorbed into the quinoa. Fluff with a fork and serve.

Curried Garbanzo Bean and Squash Stew

Dr. Cobi Slater shared this hearty stew recipe. Packed with fiber and flavor, it's sure to be a favorite. The kale is rich in calcium and magnesium, and the coconut oil contains medium-chain triglycerides that help burn fat.

• SERVES 2 TO 4 •

2 tablespoons virgin coconut oil or extra-virgin olive oil
1 medium onion, chopped
4 to 5 garlic cloves, crushed
2 teaspoons curry powder
1 teaspoon ground cumin
1 teaspoon ground coriander
½ teaspoon turmeric
½ teaspoon cinnamon
Pinch cayenne pepper
2 cups diced zucchini
2 cups diced tomatoes, or one 14-ounce can
3 to 4 cups chopped kale or spinach (if you're using kale,
    be sure to de-stem it first)
3 cups cooked garbanzo beans, or 2 cans
1 cup bean cooking liquid or water
1 to 2 teaspoons sea salt or Herbamare

Heat an 11-inch skillet or 6-quart pot over medium heat. Add the coconut oil, then the onions; sauté for about 15 minutes, or until soft. Add the crushed garlic and spices; sauté for 1 minute more. Add the zucchini and tomatoes, place the lid on the pot, and simmer over low to medium-low heat until the squash is tender, about 15 minutes. Add the chopped kale, cooked garbanzo beans, bean cooking liquid, and sea salt; gently stir together, and simmer for an additional 5 minutes. Taste and add more salt and seasoning if desired. Serve over quinoa or black rice.

Salmon Parcels

Simple, elegant, and delicious, you'll love these salmon parcels, courtesy of my friend Dr. Coby Slater. It's the perfect meal-in-a-pinch recipe. The anti-inflammatory Omega 3s found in salmon make it a great dish for any of the detoxes.

• SERVES 4 •

2 cups trimmed green beans
4 wild salmon fillets (skin on)
1 tablespoon extra-virgin olive oil
3 lemons, halved
Sea salt
Pepper

Preheat the oven to 400°. Cut 4 sheets of aluminum foil. For each piece of foil, put a handful of beans in the middle, lay a salmon fillet on top, drizzle with olive oil, squeeze half of a lemon over the top, and season with salt and pepper. Fold up aluminum foil to seal the packets, and place on a baking sheet. Cook for 15 minutes. Remove from the oven, and serve with lemon wedges. Serve with quinoa, black rice, or a side salad.

DESSERTS

Chia Breakfast Tapioca

Packed with anti-inflammatory and skin-soothing chia seeds, this alternative to the overly sweet kind makes a delicious breakfast or dessert. Courtesy Dr. Cobi Slater.

• SERVES 1 •

2 tablespoons whole white or gray chia seeds
½ cup almond milk or coconut milk (unsweetened)

Stevia to taste
Handful fresh blueberries

Place the chia seeds in a small bowl, and add the almond milk. Stir well to try to submerge most of the seeds. Allow it to sit for 20 to 30 minutes, stirring once after about 5 minutes to prevent clumping. You'll notice the seeds and liquid thickening. Stir again before serving. Makes one serving. Add stevia to taste, sprinkle a few blueberries on top, and enjoy.

You can also mix the chia and liquid, cover, and refrigerate overnight for a soft breakfast pudding the next morning.

Pumpkin Spice Drop Cookies

Cookies on a detox?!?! Seriously. On the Weekend Wonder Detox you can enjoy these delicious cookies created by Dr. Cobi Slater. They are rich in fiber, Omega 3 fatty acids, and spices that ward off bacteria and viruses.

• SERVES 10 TO 12 •

2 cups almond flour
½ cup coconut flour
1 cup chopped walnuts
½ cup organic shredded coconut
2 tablespoons powdered stevia or 20 drops liquid stevia
2 teaspoons cinnamon
1 teaspoon allspice
1 teaspoon ginger
1 teaspoon nutmeg
1 teaspoon baking soda
1 cup organic canned pumpkin
½ cup unsweetened almond milk
2 tablespoons coconut oil
3 large eggs, gently beaten
1 tablespoon grated lemon zest

Preheat oven to 375°. Line a baking sheet with parchment paper.

Mix the almond flour and next 9 ingredients (through baking soda) in a large bowl; set aside.

In a medium bowl, whisk the pumpkin, almond milk, oil, eggs, and lemon zest. Add the wet mixture to the dry mixture, and fold in until mixed. If the dough is too stiff, add a few more splashes of almond milk. The dough should not be stiff but easy to fold. Bake for 15 to 20 minutes or until lightly browned. The cookies should last about 4 days, or longer if freezing.

Thyroid-Boosting Chocolate Truffles

These chocolate truffles are packed with thyroid-boosting medium chain triglycerides and are low in sugar, making them the perfect occasional treat on the Weekend Wonder Detox.

• MAKES APPROXIMATELY 24 TRUFFLES •

1 ½ cups ground almonds
½ cup unsweetened cocoa powder (or carob powder)
½ cup coconut oil
3 fresh Medjool dates, pitted
½ teaspoon vanilla powder (Do not use vanilla sugar. Vanilla powder is
    ground vanilla beans and is available in most health food stores.)

Combine 1 cup of the ground almonds (reserve the remaining ½ cup for rolling the truffles) and all the remaining ingredients in a food processor and process until smooth. Take spoonfuls and roll into small balls, working quickly to avoid melting the coconut oil. Roll the balls into the remaining ground almonds until coated.

BODY CARE AND HOUSEHOLD PRODUCTS

Making your own body care and household products is much easier than you think, and it is a great way to avoid many harmful toxins used in commercial products.

If you can, I recommend that you keep an old blender, a small to medium glass bowl, and a spatula that you use solely for making natural aromatherapy products. Although you can use your kitchen blender, the beeswax found in natural creams can leave a residue on the blender and utensils you use.

Many of the recipes include essential oils, which are available in most health food stores. Be sure to choose essential oils, not "fragrance oil," "fragrance," or other synthetic ingredient. There are many varieties to choose from. Here is a quick overview of some of my favorites.

- Lavender essential oil is calming, eases headaches, and soothes burns or irritated skin.
- Ylang ylang is used to ease depression, insomnia, and anxiety and has a wonderful sweet smell, perfect as an alternative to perfume.
- Peppermint is uplifting, energizing, and helps with headaches.

Always start with clean utensils and blender (if using). Sterilize glass storage containers in boiling water for about ten minutes prior to adding your final products to them. Store lotions and oils in a cool place or the refrigerator. They keep for about six months but are usually used up well before that time.

Lecithin is a natural thickening agent found in most stores. It is typically derived from soy, so be sure to choose a non–genetically modified type.

Skin-Soothing Natural Body Lotion

If you're tired of all the chemicals and synthetic fragrances in most store-bought creams and lotions, consider making your own. Most people think that making creams and body lotions is difficult, but it's actually quite easy. I frequently make my own and give them as gifts to friends and family members, and they love them.

Most of the ingredients are available at your local health food store. Sweet almond oil makes a good "carrier" oil because it absorbs well and doesn't leave a greasy film. And use beeswax, as other waxes tend to be made from petroleum products. As an alternative, you can use rose water in place of the water for a decadent skin-enriching treat.

• MAKES ABOUT 2 CUPS •

¾ cup pure oil
2 tablespoons shaved beeswax
1 cup pure water
30 drops of essential oils, like lavender, ylang ylang, bergamot, or other oil
Large glass jar or 2 8-ounce glass jars for storing the lotion

Pour the oil into a Pyrex measuring cup, and add the shaved beeswax. Set the measuring cup in a saucepan of water that reaches about halfway up the side of the Pyrex container. Heat over the stove until the beeswax dissolves, and remove from the stove immediately. Allow it to cool for a minute or two but not longer than that because the beeswax will begin to harden.

Pour the water into your blender and begin blending it on high speed with the lid on (with a hole left in the lid for pouring the beeswax-oil mixture; hold a towel over the hole to prevent splashing). Slowly pour the oil-beeswax mixture into the water. It will begin to emulsify as you continue pouring the oil. It normally begins to thicken after about three-quarters of the oil has been incorporated. Continue adding the oil until you've incorporated all of it into the water.

Add the drops of essential oils you've selected; blend them into the lotion.

Pour the lotion into the glass jars you've selected for storing the cream. Use a spatula to remove any remaining lotion from the blender.

The lotion lasts for about 6 months and is best kept at cool temperatures to prolong shelf life. You can store it in the fridge if you choose to keep it fresh.

That's it! It's not as hard as you might think, and your skin and the rest of your body will thank you for giving it healing natural lotion rather than the harsh chemicals found in most creams and lotions. Enjoy!

Hormone-Balancing Massage Oil

Whether you're suffering from the effects of stress, depression, anxiety, PMS, or menopause or you're fatigued and just need a boost, this massage oil blend is ideal. Of course, I'm not talking about a caffeine sort of jolt but rather a gentle energy and emotional boost that happens with regular use. This oil also works well for women suffering from hormone-linked skin issues.

Rub this oil onto your skin after showering while your skin is still damp or before bed to help you let go of stress and worries. It can be used for any of the weekend detoxes but is particularly suited for the Colon Cleanse Weekend (for this weekend, rub it in clockwise circles on your abdomen) and the Skin Rejuvenation Weekend.

Bergamot oil helps lessen depression and anxiety. It is anti-inflammatory, to help reduce the likelihood of experiencing skin blemishes and scarring. Clary sage balances the effects of stress while also balancing women's hormones, making it perfect for this blend.

When I've got a serious case of monkey mind—I'm lying in bed, running through all the things I need to do tomorrow and what happened during the day, unable to get to sleep—I use frankincense to help me relax and let go of worries. It alleviates anxiety, stress, and depression, and it helps clear out the "cobwebs" from the mind and body. Ylang ylang helps to replenish the body when it has suffered the ravages of stress and exhaustion while also helping to balance women's hormones.

• MAKES ABOUT 8 OUNCES •

You will need the following ingredients. Don't worry if you can't find all of the essential oils or if you can only afford a couple—they'll still have powerful emotional and physical healing effects.

8 ounces sweet almond oil
7 drops bergamot essential oil
10 drops clary sage essential oil
3 drops frankincense essential oil

30 drops ylang ylang

Small to medium brown or cobalt blue glass bottle with a lid

Fill a sterilized, brown glass bottle with the 8 ounces of sweet almond oil.

Add the drops of essential oils. Cover with the lid and gently roll the bottle between your palms to mix thoroughly. It's ready for use.

Skin-Soothing Chapped Skin Ointment

This natural, soothing, and healing ointment is great for dry skin and chapped lips or hands, and it is perfect for healing rashes or skin irritations. It is surprisingly simple to make and better than store-bought skin care products, which are replete with synthetic and toxic preservatives as well as other additives.

Small pot

1 cup of pure cold-pressed oil, such as olive, almond, hazelnut,
    grape seed, or avocado

1 tablespoon beeswax

10 drops of your favorite essential oils, such as lavender, ylang ylang,
    or peppermint

30 drops pure carrot essential oil (optional)

3 4-ounce sterilized glass jars with lids

In a small pot, over low heat on the stove, combine oil, beeswax, and all essential oils. Slowly heat until the beeswax is melted. Do not let ingredients boil, as heat damages the integrity of the oils—it is best to work slowly.

Whisk or stir ingredients to be sure they are blended, and pour into glass jars (available at many natural food stores). Let sit until cool. Store in a cool place. Will store for about 1 year.

OPTION: Congestion-Soothing Chest Rub: In place of the carrot oil use eucalyptus essential oil to create a soothing vaporizing chest rub to ease sinus and lung congestion. For this recipe you can omit the other essential oils and just use eucalyptus.

Natural Toothpaste

Most toothpaste contains sugar, fluoride, artificial colors, and other harmful ingredients that are best avoided. Instead of using the toxic commercial varieties, why not make your own? It's simple and quick. Once you have the essential oils needed, you can use them to make the toothpaste or, rather, tooth powder, which more accurately describes it, for years to come.

The peppermint essential oil helps freshen breath, kill bacteria, and clear sinuses. The myrrh oil is highly antibacterial and antifungal. The baking soda restores a natural, slightly alkaline pH balance to the teeth and gums.

• MAKES ABOUT ½ CUP •

½ cup baking soda
10 drops pure peppermint essential oil (this is not the same as
        peppermint extract or fragrance oil. Also, it should be a
        high-quality food-grade essential oil, which is available from
        many health food stores)
5 drops pure myrrh essential oil (optional)

Mix all ingredients in a small jar with a lid, cover, and shake well to disperse oils throughout. Use a small amount on a damp toothbrush the way you would use toothpaste. Store in a covered jar for about 3 months.

Aromatherapy Facial Cream

This natural aromatherapy facial cream is easy to make and perfect for dry or problem skin, particularly hormonally linked problem skin.

• MAKES ENOUGH TO FILL ABOUT 3 8-OUNCE JARS •

6 ounces organic sweet almond oil
2 ounces organic avocado oil (if you can't find avocado oil, you can
        substitute more sweet almond oil)
¾ cup shaved beeswax (use a grater)

I teaspoon lecithin granules

I cup lukewarm water

Essential oils

10 drops chamomile

6 drops eucalyptus

2 drops frankincense

20 drops lavender

2 drops patchouli

10 drops ylang ylang

Equipment

Blender

Pyrex container, sterilized

Double boiler

You can use a different combination of the essential oils if you prefer. Use about 30 to 50 total drops of either a single oil or combined essential oils.

Measure the sweet almond and avocado oil into a sterilized Pyrex container. Add the shaved beeswax. Bring a double boiler filled with water to a boil. Set the Pyrex container in the box, gently warming the oil and beeswax mixture until the beeswax is melted. Remove immediately from the stove. In a separate bowl, dilute the lecithin granules in the cup of lukewarm purified water. Pour the water-lecithin mixture into the blender, and begin blending. Slowly add the oil mixture, blending until the mixture forms a cream. Finally, add the essential oils; blend until combined. Immediately fill sterilized glass jars and label. The cream lasts about 6 months when kept refrigerated.

Emotional Support with Bach Flower Remedies

Sometimes emotions can come up when detoxifying. If you are suffering from exhaustion, loneliness, fear, or uncertainty, Bach flower therapy may be helpful. British medical doctor and bacteriologist Dr. Edward Bach founded a system of treating emotional imbalances using the "essence" of flowers. He carefully studied and developed remedies from wild flowers to work on mental fixations and emotions that may be producing harmful effects on the body.

Many homeopaths, doctors of natural medicine, and other natural health practitioners practice Bach flower therapy. The basic principle is simple: people with fearful, worried, or depressed mental states tend to heal slower and less completely than do those with positive, cheerful, and hopeful states of mind.

It can be a bit confusing, though, with almost forty remedies to choose from. Here are four of my emotional detox remedies to help you get started. I've included information to take them with water, but you can also add four drops to a bathtub as well. Bach flower essences or remedies are available in most health food stores or online at bachflower.com.

Overworked and Worn Out: Olive

Our fast-paced life can take its toll on our energy. If you're exhausted from balancing work, home, and personal demands, Olive is the remedy to help you regenerate body, mind, and spirit. It is the remedy of choice when you are exhausted from excessive work demands or are suffering from a lack of sleep. Add 2 to 4 drops of Olive to a glass of water 4 times daily for several weeks or until you start feeling greater vitality.

Depressed and Unhappy: Wild Rose

Do you feel stuck in your life, depressed that life hasn't gone the way you wanted or are simply unhappy with your circumstances? The Bach Flower Remedy Wild Rose is the one to choose when you feel a lack of joy in life, are bored with your current circumstances, derive no satisfaction from your achievements, or feel like you're stuck in a holding pattern. Add 2 to 4 drops to a glass of water 4 times daily until you feel like life holds more joy and excitement.

Adjusting to Life Changes: Walnut

Regardless of whether you're starting a new job, moving away, experiencing menopause, leaving a long-term relationship, or retiring, Walnut is the remedy to help you adjust to new life circumstances. It also helps if you know you need to make a change and just don't think you have the courage or resolve to do so. Take 2 to 4 drops in a glass of water 4 times daily during major or minor life changes.

Traumatized, Injured, or Stressed Out: Rescue Remedy

If you're dealing with traumas, injuries, serious stresses, or just don't know which remedy to choose, Rescue Remedy is the flower essence to select. It contains five flower essences: Star of Bethlehem for trauma and shock, Rock Rose for terror and panic, Impatiens for irritability and tension, Cherry Plum for fear of losing control, and Clematis for being more emotionally present in life. Rescue Remedy is suitable for physical or emotional traumas, injuries, or simply to help you through difficult experiences. Like the other remedies, take 2 to 4 drops of Rescue Remedy in a glass of water 4 times daily for as long as necessary.

Of course, you should always consult a physician or other qualified health professional if you're experiencing ongoing emotional troubles or depression.

ABOUT THE AUTHOR

Michelle Schoffro Cook is the author of fifteen health books, including the international bestsellers: *60 Seconds to Slim*, *The Ultimate pH Solution*, and *The 4-Week Ultimate Body Detox Plan*. She holds advanced degrees in natural health, holistic and orthomolecular nutrition, and has over twenty years of experience in the field. She is the publisher of the popular health e-zine *World's Healthiest News* and is a regular blogger for HealthySurvivalist.com and Care2.com. Check out her websites: DrMichelleCook.com and WorldsHealthiestDiet.com. Subscribe to her free e-zine at www.WorldsHealthiestDiet.com.

ACKNOWLEDGMENTS

Thank you to Renée for your belief in this book and for your approachable, down-to-earth, friendly style. You're a joy to work with and a lovely person.

Thank you to the team at Da Capo for all your efforts on design, editing, marketing, and promotions to make *Weekend Wonder Detox* what it is and what it will become.

Anita Santos, thanks for being a beautiful fitness model and wonderful friend.

To my wonderful agent and good friend, Claire. You're a visionary and a great agent. Thanks for all your efforts.

To my amazing husband—the love of my life and my soul mate—I cannot thank you enough for all you do for me.

To my parents, Michael and Deborah Schoffro. Thanks for believing in me since I was a child.

To Maria Yarek, thanks for the great photography.

Thanks to everyone else who played a role in this book.

RESOURCES

More Information About Dr. Michelle Schoffro Cook

World's Healthiest News

Subscribe to Dr. Schoffro Cook's free e-zine *World's Healthiest News* to get the latest natural health insights, news, research, recipes, and more. Each edition features concise information you can immediately use to boost your energy, enhance detoxification, supercharge your immune system, look great, and feel great. You'll find delicious and nutritious recipes as well as cutting-edge research on nutrition, disease prevention, and healing. You'll also get exclusive deals on some of your favorite health products and discover health tips that you can apply to your life today, all from a source you can trust and at a price you can't beat—FREE! Subscribe at www.WorldsHealthiestDiet.com.

Dr. Schoffro Cook's Blogs

Follow Dr. Schoffro Cook's popular blogs:

www.DrMichelleCook.com
www.HealthySurvivalist.com
www.probioticmiracle.com
www.care2.com/greenliving/author/mcook

Genetically Modified Foods

Dr. Schoffro Cook regularly discusses genetically modified foods in her blogs and e-zine. In addition, she recommends the following books and website for more information on this important topic:

Seeds of Deception: Exposing Industry and Government Lies About the Safety of Genetically Engineered Foods by Jeffrey M. Smith (Yes! Books, 2003)

Genetic Roulette: The Documented Health Risks of Genetically Engineered Foods by Jeffrey M. Smith (Yes! Books, 2007)

Seeds of Deception, www.seedsofdeception.com

Water Filtration

There are many different types of water filtration systems, including activated carbon (such as Brita makes), reverse osmosis, ultraviolet (UV) systems, distillation, water ionizers, and water alkalinizers. They vary greatly in terms of the toxins they remove from water. Here's a brief overview:

Activated carbon can absorb thousands of different toxic compounds. These filtration systems are available in under-the-counter models, pitchers, and water bottles.

Reverse osmosis is highly effective against bacteria, viruses, arsenic, fluoride, nitrates, and most of the substances captured by activated carbon.

Ultraviolet (UV) light is a form of radiation that kills viruses, mold, algae, bacteria, and yeasts; however, it doesn't work well against heavy metals. As a result it is often combined with other forms of filtration.

Distillation removes all minerals, including beneficial ones from water. Although many health practitioners love distilled water, I'm not a fan. I feel it is essentially "dead" and may leach minerals out of the body. However, it is highly effective against heavy metals.

Ionization is a means of adding negative ions to water to enable it to neutralize toxins (as they tend to have a positive electrical charge). Proponents claim that it renders the water more usable by the body's cells, allowing faster rehydration.

For specific brand recommendations and deals on some of my favorite water filtration systems, subscribe to my free e-zine *World's Healthiest News* at my website: www.DrMichelleCook.com.

Herb Suppliers

There are many excellent companies offering dried, bulk herbs or herbal tinctures. They include:

Aroma Borealis
www.aromaborealis.com

Harmonic Arts
www.harmonicarts.ca

Mountain Rose Herbs
www.mountainroseherbs.com

Beauty Ingredients

There are thousands of toxic ingredients used in beauty products. I regularly write about them on my blogs; please be sure to check them out. Additionally, here are some sites that offer more information about cosmetic ingredients:

The Campaign for Safe Cosmetics
www.safecosmetics.org

EWG's Skin Deep Cosmetics Database
www.ewg.org/skindeep

NOTES

Chapter 1: Why You Need to Detox

1. Jenny L. Carwile and Karin B. Michels, "Urinary Bisphenol A and Obesity: NHANES 2003–2006," *Environmental Research* 111, no. 6 (August 2011): 825–830, www.ncbi.nlm.nih.gov/pubmed/21676388.

2. Diana I. Jalal, Gerard Smits, Richard J. Johnson, and Michel Chonchol, "Increased Fructose Associates with Elevated Blood Pressure," *Journal of the American Society of Nephrology* 21, no. 9 (September 2010): 1543–1549, www.ncbi.nlm.nih.gov/pubmed/20595676.

3. Betty Kovacs, "Artificial Sweeteners: Health and Disease Prevention," MedicineNet, www.onhealth.com/artificial_sweeteners/page6 .htm.

4. Joseph Mercola, "Health Risks of Genetically Modified Foods," Mercola, http://articles.mercola.com/sites/articles/archive/2008/01/02 /health-risks-of-genetically-modified-foods.aspx.

5. Joseph Mercola, "19 Studies Link GMO Foods to Organ Disruption," Mercola, April 27, 2011, http://articles.mercola.com/sites/articles /archive/2011/04/27/19-studies-link-gmo-foods-to-organ-disruption.aspx.

Chapter 2: Getting Ready to Detox

1. Mette Kristensen, Marlene Jensen, Jane Kudsk, Marianne Henriksen, and Christian Molgaard, "Short-Term Effects on Bone Turnover of Replacing Milk with Cola Beverages: A 10-Day Interventional Study in Young Men," *Osteoporosis International* 16, no. 2 (December 2005): 1803–1808; S. Johnson, "Multifaceted and Widespread Pathology of

Magnesium Deficiency," *Medical Hypotheses* 56, no. 2 (February 2001): 163–170; K. L. Tucker, K. Morita, N. Qiao, M. T. Hannan, L. A. Cupples, and D. P Kiel, "Colas, but Not Other Carbonated Beverages, Are Associated with Low Bone Mineral Density in Older Women: The Framingham Osteoporosis Study," *American Journal of Clinical Nutrition* 84, no. 2 (October 2006): 936–942; G. Wykshak and R. E. Frisch, "Carbonated Beverages, Dietary Calcium, the Dietary Calcium/Phosphorus Ratio, and Bone Fractures in Girls and Boys," *Journal of Adolescent Health* 15, no. 3 (May 1994): 210–215.

2. "Sprouting," Wikipedia, http://en.wikipedia.org/wiki/Sprouting.

3. Ibid.

4. Ibid.

5. Ibid.

Chapter 3: The Love Your Liver Weekend

1. Frances Albrecht, "The Basics of Detoxing Your Liver," *Healthwell*, April 1997.

2. Scott Rigden, "Liver Detoxification," www.drscottrigden.com. See also Michelle Schoffro Cook, *The 4-Week Ultimate Body Detox Plan: A Program for Greater Energy, Health and Vitality* (Toronto: Wiley, 2006), 223–224.

3. "Avocado," The World's Healthiest Foods, www.whfoods.com/gen page.php?tname=foodspice&dbid=5.

4. "Fat-Burning Foods," *Woman's World*, April 27, 2004.

5. Ann Louise Gittleman, *The Fat Flush Plan* (New York: McGraw-Hill, 2002), 19.

6. Michael Murray, *Dr. Murray's Total Body Tune-Up* (New York: Bantam Books, 2000), 78.

7. Xandria Williams, *The Herbal Detox Plan* (Carlsbad, CA: Hay House, 2003), 129.

8. Robert Bentely and Henry Trimen, *Medicinal Plants*, vol. 3 (London: J & A Churchill, 1880), 159.

9. K. Faber, "The Dandelion—Taraxacum Officinale Weber," *Pharmazie* 13, no. 7 (July 1958), 423–435.

10. A. Mahesh, R. Jeyachandran, L. Cindrella, D. Thanqadurai, V. P. Veerapur, and D. Muralidhara Rao, "Hepatocurative Potential of Sesquiterpene Lactones of Taraxacum Officinale on Carbon Tetrachloride Induced Liver Toxicity in Mice," *Acta Biologica Hungarica* 61, No. 2 (June 2010): 175–190, http://www.ncbi.nlm.nih.gov/pubmed/20519172.

11. Albrecht, "The Basics of Detoxing Your Liver."

Chapter 4: The Lymphomania Weekend

1. Michelle Schoffro Cook, "The Secret of Great Health: An Interview with Best-Selling Author Harvey Diamond," April 2003.

2. Jillian Boyle, "Is Lymphatic Stress the Reason You're Fat? Bloated? Hungry for Junk Food?" *Woman's World*, March 2, 2004.

3. Ann Louise Gittleman, *The Fat Flush Plan* (New York: McGraw-Hill, 2002), 21.

4. Michelle Schoffro Cook, *The 4-Week Ultimate Body Detox Plan* (Toronto: Wiley, 2004).

Chapter 5: The Kidney Flush Weekend

1. Gary Null, with Amy McDonald, *Be a Healthy Woman!* (New York: Seven Stories Press, 2009), 608.

2. Ann Louise Gittleman, *The Fat Flush Plan* (New York: McGraw-Hill, 2002), 27.

3. M. E. El-Mesery, M. M. Al-Gayyar, H. A. Salem, M. M. Darweish, and A. M. El-Mowafy, "Chemopreventive and Renal Protective Effects for Docosahexaenoic Acid (DHA): Implications of CRP and Lipid Peroxides," *Cell Division* 4, no. 1 (April 2009): 6, www.ncbi.nlm.nih.gov/pubmed/19341447.

4. M. Twal, P. Kiefer, A. Salameh, J. Schnabel, S. Ossmann, S. von Salisch, K. Kramer, et. al., "Reno-Protective Effects of Epigallocatechingallate in a Small Piglet Model of Extracorporeal Circulation," *Pharmacological Research* 67, no. 1 (January 2013): 68–8, www.ncbi.nlm.nih.gov/pubmed/23103594; A. M. El-Mowafy, H. A. Salem, M. M. Al-Gayyar, M. E. El-Mesery, and M. F. El-Azab, "Evaluation of Renal Protective Effects of the Green-Tea (EGCG) and Red Grape Resveratrol: Role of Oxidative Stress and Inflammatory Cytokines," *Natural Product Research* 25, no. 8 (April 2011): 850–856, www.ncbi.nlm.nih.gov/pubmed/21462079.

5. El-Mowafy, et al., "Evaluation of Renal Protective Effects of the Green-Tea (EGCG) and Red Grape Resveratrol."

6. Jyh-Gang Leu, Chin-Yao Lin, Jhin-Hao Jian, Chin-Yu Shih, Yao-Jen Liang, "Epigallocatechin-3-Gallate Combined with Alpha Lipoic Acid Attenuates High Glucose-Induced Receptor for Advanced Glycation End Products (RAGE) Expression in Human Embryonic Kidney Cells," *Anais da Academia Brasileira de Ciências* 85, no. 2 (June 2013): 745–752, www.ncbi.nlm.nih.gov/pubmed/23780308.

7. Anurag Kuhad, Sangeeta Pilkhwal, Sameer Sharma, Naveen Tirkey, and Kanwaljit Chopra, "Effect of Curcumin on Inflammation and

Oxidative Stress in Cisplatin-Induced Experimental Nephrotoxicity," *Journal of Agricultural Food Chemistry* 55, no. 25 (December 2007): 10150–10155, www.ncbi.nlm.nih.gov/pubmed/23780308.

8. M. A. Beerepoot, G. ter Riet, S. Nys, W. M. vad der Wal, C. A. de Borgie, T. M. de Reijke, J. M. Prins, et. al., "Lactobacilli vs. Antibiotics to Prevent Urinary Tract Infections: A Randomized, Double-Blind, Non-inferiority Trial in Postmenopausal Women," *Archives of Internal Medicine* 172, no. 9 (May 2012): 704–712, www.ncbi.nlm.nih.gov/pubmed /22782199.

9. Joseph Mercola, "Six Ways to Keep Kidney Stones at Bay," Mercola.com, September 29, 2011, http://articles.mercola.com/sites/articles /archive/2011/09/29/six-ways-to-keep-kidney-stones-at-bay-from-the -harvard-health-letter.aspx.

10. Leu, et al., "Epigallocatechin-3-Gallate Combined with Alpha Lipoic Acid Attenuates High Glucose-Induced Receptor."

11. Ilchi Lee, *Meridian Exercise for Self-Healing* (Sedona, AZ: BEST Life Media, 2008), 97, 230–231.

Chapter 6: The Colon Cleanse Weekend

1. Patricia Fitzgerald, *The Detox Solution: The Missing Link to Radiant Health, Abundant Energy, Ideal Weight, and Peace of Mind* (Santa Monica, CA: Illumination Press, 2001), 140.

2. Ibid.

3. Xandria Williams, *The Herbal Detox Plan: The Revolutionary Way to Cleanse and Revive Your Body* (Carlsbad, CA: Hay House, 2004), 83; Gloria Gilbère, "A Doctor's Solution to 'Plumbing Problems,' in Your Gut That Is!" *Total Health* 26, no. 1 (February 2004), 37.

Chapter 7: The Skin Rejuvenation Weekend

1. Shari Lieberman and Nancy Bruning, *The Real Vitamin & Mineral Book: The Definitive Guide to Designing Your Personal Supplement Program* (New York: Avery, 2003), 91.

Chapter 8: The Fat Blast Weekend

1. Kevin Gianni, "7 of the Most Unhealthy and Potentially Cancer-Causing Foods," *Renegade Health*, May 21, 2012, http://renegadehealth

.com/blog/2012/05/21/7-of-the-most-unhealthy-and-potentially-cancer
-causing-foods.

2. "How Many Pounds Does One Extra Soft Drink Add to Your Body?" Mercola.com, August 24, 2006, http://articles.mercola.com/sites/articles/archive/2006/08/24/how-many-pounds-does-one-extra-soft-drink-add-to-your-body.aspx.

3. Robert Crayhon, "The Ultimate Weight Loss Nutrient," *Total Health Resource Guide: Healthy Weight Management,* July/August 2002, 12.

4. S. Rayalam, M. A. Della-Fara, J. Y. Yang, H. J. Park, S. Ambati, C. Baile "Resveratrol Potentiates Genistein's Antiadipogenic and Pro-Apoptotic Effects in 3T3-L1 Adipocytes," *Journal of Nutrition* 137, no. 12 (December 2007): 2668–2673, www.ncbi.nlm.nih.gov/pubmed/18029481.

5. A. Bhattacharya, M. M. Rahman, R. McCarter, M. O'Shea, and G. Fernandes, "Conjugated Linoleic Acid and Chromium Lower Body Weight and Visceral Fat Mass in High-Fat-Diet-Fed Mice," *Lipids* 41, no. 5 (May 2006): 437–444, www.ncbi.nlm.nih.gov/pubmed/16933788.

6. Bernard Gout, Cédric Bourges, and Séverine Paineau-Dubreuil, "Satiereal, a Crocus sativus L. Extract, Reduces Snacking and Increases Satiety in a Randomized, Placebo-Controlled Study of Mildly Overweight, Healthy Women," *Nutrition Research* 30, no. 5 (May 2010): 305–313, www.ncbi.nlm.nih.gov/pubmed/20579522.

7. Akira Niijima and Katsuya Nagai, "Effect of Olfactory Stimulation with Flavor of Grapefruit Oil and Lemon Oil on the Activity of Sympathetic Branch in the White Adipose Tissue of the Epididymis," *Experimental Biological Medicine* 228, no. 10 (November 2003): 1190–1192.

INDEX

Acetone, 27

Acne, 174–75, 179

Acrylamide, 210

Acupressure
abdominal massage, 162–164
for kidney detox and healing, 135–137
for liver detox and healing, 83–85

Additives, MSG in, 19–20

Air fresheners, 27–28

Almonds
for skin rejuvenation, 181
Thyroid-Boosting Chocolate Truffles, 268

Aloe vera, 159

Alpha lipoic acid (ALA), 129–130

AminoSweet, 11–13, 211

Ammonia, 119

Appetizers, Dips, and Spreads
Better Than Butter, 250
Chickpea Bread, 251–252
Chili Lime Green Beans, 252
Dairy-Free Yogurt, 248–249
Herbes de Provence Cashew Cheese, 250–251
Lemon-Garlic Greens, 252–253
Portobello Mushroom Gravy, 253–254
Sweet Potato Fries, 249

Arachidonic acid, 42

Aromatherapy abdominal massage, 223–226

Aromatherapy compress, 85–86

Aromatherapy Facial Cream, 273–274

Aromatherapy skin softener bath, 189–190

Arthritis, 41

Artificial sweeteners, 11–16, 39–40, 211

Aspartame, 11–13, 211

Astragalus
for lymph detox, 104
Lymphomania Herbal Tea, 245

Avocados, 73–74, 181

Baby food, 18

Bach, Edward, 274–275

Bach flower essences, 275

Back pain, 118–119

Bacon, 210

Bacteria, intestinal, 148–149

Baths, therapeutic, 189–190

Bean(s)
  Chickpea Bread, 251–252
  for detox weekends, 53–54
  for Fat Blast Weekend, 212
  Garbanzo, and Squash Stew,
    Curried, 265
  Green, Chili Lime, 252
  Roasted Red Pepper Chickpea
    Mash, 263
  Salmon Parcels, 266
Bearberry
  for kidney detox, 130–131
  Kidney Herbal Tea, 246
Beets
  for liver detox, 74
  Liver Jumpstart Juice, 242
  Weekend Wonder Detox
    Signature Salad, 258–259
Benzene, 26, 28
Bergamot oil, 271
Berries. See also Cranberry(ies)
  Chia Breakfast Tapioca,
    266–267
  for colon cleanse, 154–155
  for skin rejuvenation, 181, 182
Beverages. See also Green Tea; Tea
  buying fruits and vegetables
    for, 239
  Cantaloupe Ice, 241
  Carrot Celery Juice, 240
  Celery Cucumber Juice, 240
  Citrus Boost, 241–242
  Cranberry Pear Juice, 242
  Cucumber Mint Refresh, 240
  fruit juices, in detox weekends,
    125, 179, 205
  juicers for, 239
  Liver Jumpstart Juice, 242
  Mom's Energy Smoothie, 244
  vegetable juices, in detox
    weekends, 125, 178–179,
    204, 205
  Watermelon Ice, 241

Bifidobacteria, 149, 157
Bisphenol-A (BPA), 7
Black cohosh, 187
Bladder tumors, 14
Blaylock, Russell, 19
Blood sugar, 205–206, 212
Blueberries
  Chia Breakfast Tapioca,
    266–267
  for skin rejuvenation, 181
Body care products
  Aromatherapy Facial Cream,
    273–274
  clogged skin pores from, 176
  homemade, preparing,
    268–269
  Hormone-Balancing Massage Oil,
    271–272
  natural, switching to, 180
  Natural Toothpaste, 273
  Skin-Soothing Chapped Skin
    Ointment, 272
  Skin-Soothing Natural Body
    Lotion, 269–270
  store-bought, ingredients in,
    22–25
  toxins in, 22–25, 174–175, 176,
    177–178, 180
Brain health, 149
Brain tumors, 13
Bread, Chickpea, 251–252
Breakouts, 174–175
Breast disease, 148
Brown rice
  about, 43–44
  Spicy, Rice-y Detox Soup,
    260–261
Buchu
  for kidney detox, 131
  Kidney Herbal Tea, 246
Buckwheat, 44
Butane, 27
Butter, Better Than, 250

Caffeine withdrawal, 64
Cancer
    and agricultural pesticides, 48
    and aspartame, 13
    and bowel movements, 148
    and environment, 3
    and food colors, 8
    and processed meats, 210
Canola, 22, 180
Cantaloupe, for skin
        rejuvenation, 181
Cantaloupe Ice, 241
Carnitine, 214
Carrot(s)
    Celery Juice, 240
    Liver Jumpstart Juice, 242
    Weekend Wonder Detox
        Signature Salad, 258–259
Cascara sagrada
    for colon cleanse, 159
    Colon Cleanse Herbal Tea,
        246–247
Cayenne, 212
Celery Carrot Juice, 240
Celery Cucumber Juice, 240
Cellulite, 97
Chest presses, 220
Chia Breakfast Tapioca, 266–267
Chickpea Bread, 251–252
Chloroform, 26
Chocolate Truffles, Thyroid-
        Boosting, 268
Chromium, 215–216, 217–218
Chronic fatigue syndrome
        (CFS), 68
Cinnamon, 213
Clary sage oil, 271
Cleaning products, 25–26
Cleavers
    for kidney detox, 131
    Kidney Herbal Tea, 246
    for lymph detox, 104–105
    Lymphomania Herbal Tea, 245

    for skin rejuvenation, 186–187
    Skin Rejuvenation Herbal Tea, 247
Coal tar, 24
Coconut
    Pumpkin Spice Drop Cookies,
        267–268
    Vegetable Soup, Thai, 261–262
Coconut oil
    Better Than Butter, 250
    cooking with, 55
Colon Cleanse Weekend, 145–171
    benefits of, 145–147
    conclusion of, 166
    critical nutrients, 157–158
    dietary suggestions, 149–156
    exercises, 160–162
    grocery list, 167–168
    herbal cleansers, 158–160
    journal, 168–171
    reasons for detox, 147–149
    signs of intestinal imbalances, 150
    spa treatments, 162–164
    weekend schedule, 164–166
    worksheets, 167–171
Conjugated linoleic acid (CLA),
        215–216
Constipation, 148
Cookies, Pumpkin Spice Drop,
        267–268
Corn, genetically-modified, 21, 209
Corn chips, 209
Corn sweetener, 10
Corn syrup, 10
Cosmetics, toxins in, 177–178
Cottonseed oil, 22
Cranberry(ies)
    Green Tea Lemonade, 243–244
    for kidney detox, 122, 125–126
    for lymph detox, 100
    Pear Juice, 242
Cranberry juice, 100, 122, 125–126
Crane Pose, 82–83
Cravings, eliminating, 217–218

Croutons, salad, 18
Cucumber(s)
    Celery Juice, 240
    Cucumber-Mint Salad, 258
    Liver Jumpstart Juice, 242
    Mint Refresh, 240
    Curcumin, 81–82, 127
Curls, 220
Curried Garbanzo Bean and
    Squash Stew, 265
Cytokines, 149

Dairy products, avoiding, 40–41,
    99, 207
Dandelion greens
    for kidney detox, 131–132
    for liver detox, 74
    Liver Jumpstart Juice, 242
Dandelion root
    Kidney Herbal Tea, 246
    for liver detox, 80–81
    Love Your Liver Herbal Tea,
    244–245
Dehydration, 119–120, 218
Deodorizers, 27–28
Depression, 275
Desserts
    Chia Breakfast Tapioca, 266–267
    Pumpkin Spice Drop Cookies,
    267–268
    Thyroid-Boosting Chocolate
    Truffles, 268
Detox weekends
    after the weekend ends, 64,
    235–237
    compared with dieting, 62
    comparing detox programs, 63
    drinking water during, 48–50
eating small meals during, 56
    exercises and spa treatments,
    58–60
    foods to avoid, 38–43
    frequently asked questions, 61–64

gluten-free grains for, 43–45
health benefits, 2–6, 61
herbs for, 57–58
legumes, nuts, and seeds for,
    53–54
multivitamin and minerals for,
    56–57
negative symptoms during,
    63–64
nondairy milk for, 55
oils and spices for, 55–56
organic foods for, 46–48
quiz, for identifying symptoms,
    31–37
safety of, 61–62
salads and vegetables for, 51–52
side effects from, 63
sprouts and fruit for, 52–53
Dextrose, 10
Diabetes, 9
Diamond, Harvey, 95
Diazolidinyl urea, 23
Dibutyl phthalate, 26
Dieting, 62
Dioxins, 24
Docosahexaenoic acid (DHA),
    123–24, 126, 181
Dong quai, 187
Doughnuts, 211
Dry skin brushing, 108–109
Dyes, 8, 23

Echinacea
    for lymph detox, 104
    Lymphomania Herbal Tea, 245
EGCG (epigallocatechin gallate),
    126, 212, 216
Eggs, 74
Emotional detox remedies, 274–276
Entrées
    Curried Garbanzo Bean and
    Squash Stew, 265
    Ginger Chili Quinoa, 264

Lentil Bowl, 263–264
Roasted Red Pepper Chickpea
    Mash, 263
Salmon Parcels, 266
Veggie Scramble, 262–263
Enzymes, 41, 52
Essential fatty acids, 52
Ethyl parabens, 23
Exercises
cardiovascular, 160–161,
    187–188, 219
Crane Pose, 82–83
enjoyable, choosing, 203
knees to chest, 161–162
leg sweep and swing, 132–133
rebounding, 105–106
strength training, 219–223

Fabric softeners, 24
Fat Blast Weekend, 201–233
benefits of, 201–203
conclusion of, 228
critical nutrients, 213–216
curing sugar cravings, 217–218
dietary suggestions, 203–213
exercises, 219–223
grocery list, 229–230
herbs that burn fat, 216–217
journal, 230–233
spa treatments, 223–226
weekend schedule, 226–228
worksheets, 229–233
Fats, dietary, 16–17, 179–180, 211
Fatty liver, 70
Feminine hygiene products, 24
Fiber, 151, 153–156
Fiber supplements, 157
Fibromyalgia, 68, 96
Fish
chemicals and pesticides in, 7, 43
for detox weekends, 42–43
for kidney detox, 123–124, 126
Omega 3s in, 42–43

Salmon Parcels, 266
for skin rejuvenation, 181
Flax seeds / flax seed oil
Better Than Butter, 250
for colon cleanse, 157
for Fat Blast Weekend, 213
for liver detox, 74–75
for lymph detox, 101
Mom's Energy Smoothie, 244
for skin rejuvenation, 182, 185
Flower therapy, 274–276
Fluoride, 24
Food colors, 8
Food labels, 10, 11, 19–20
Formaldehyde, 23, 26, 28
Fragrances, 24
Frankincense oil, 271
French fries, 209–210
Fructose, 10
Fruit. *See also specific fruits*
avoiding sugar cravings with, 218
buying, for juices, 239
for colon cleanse, 151
for detox weekends, 40, 53
juices, for detox weekends, 125,
    179, 205
for liver detox, 72
for lymph detox, 99–100
Mom's Energy Smoothie, 244
weight gain from, 40, 53

Garlic
for Fat Blast Weekend, 212
Garlic-Lemon Greens, 252–253
for liver detox, 75
Gastrointestinal tract (GI),
    147–149
Genetically modified organisms
    (GMOs), 20–22, 46
Ginger Chili Quinoa, 264
Globe artichoke, 81
Glutathione, 77–78
Gluten, 43–45, 151

GMOs. *See* Genetically modified
   organisms
Grains, 43–45, 155
Grapefruit
   Citrus Boost, 241–242
   Citrus Power Dressing, 260
Grape seed extract, 215
Green Beans
   Chili Lime, 252
   Salmon Parcels, 266
Green powder
   about, 239
   Mom's Energy Smoothie, 244
Greens
   bitter, phytochemicals in, 71–72
   for colon cleanse, 155–156
   Curried Garbanzo Bean and
      Squash Stew, 265
   dandelion, 74, 131–132
   for Fat Blast Weekend, 212
   for kidney detox, 131–132
   Lemon-Garlic, 252–253
   for liver detox, 71–72, 74, 75
   Liver Jumpstart Juice, 242
   for lymph detox, 100
   for skin rejuvenation, 182
   Weekend Wonder Detox
      Signature Salad, 258–259
Green Tea
   for caffeine withdrawals, 64
   Cranberry Lemonade, 243–244
   for Fat Blast Weekend, 212,
      216–217
   for kidney detox, 126–127
   Lemonade, Super-Detoxifying,
      243
Grocery lists, 60

Headaches, 64
Heart attack, 11
Herbes de Provence Cashew Cheese,
   250–251
Herbs, for detox weekends, 57–58

HFCS. *See* High-fructose corn syrup
High blood pressure, 11, 120, 121
High-fructose corn syrup (HFCS),
   10–11
Hives, 174–175
Honey, 8–9, 40
Honey-Turmeric Tea, 247
Hormone-Balancing Massage Oil,
   271–272
Hot dogs, 210
Hydrogenated fats, 17, 179–180

Ice cream, 209
Imidazolidinyl urea, 23
Immune system, 68, 147, 149
Infant formula, 18
Inflammation
   and gastrointestinal health, 147
   from HFCS, 11
   link to illnesses, 17
   from omega 6 fatty acids, 42
   reducing, with licorice root, 160
   reducing, with Omega 3s, 42
   waste products from, 97
Intestines. *See also* Colon Cleanse
      Weekend
   detoxifying, benefits of, 145
   function of, 147–149
Irritable bowel syndrome, 146
Isobutane, 27
Isoflavones, 214–215

Kidney Flush Weekend, 117–143
   benefits of, 117
   conclusion of, 139
   critical nutrients, 127–130
   dietary suggestions, 122–127
   exercises, 132–133
   grocery list, 140
   herbal kidney boosters, 130–132
   journal, 141–143
   reasons for detox, 117–119
   signs of stressed kidneys, 119–121

spa treatments, 134–137
weekend schedule, 137–139
worksheets, 140–143
Kidneys. *See also* Kidney Flush
Weekend
function of, 117
and kidney stones, 121
Knee lifts, 221
Knees to chest exercise, 161–162

Lactobacilli, 149, 157
Lactose, 10
Laundry products, 174–175
Lead, in cosmetics, 24
Lecithin, 78
Leg lifts, 221
Leg sweep and swing, 132–133
Legumes. *See also* Bean(s)
for colon cleanse, 153
for detox weekends, 53–54
for Fat Blast Weekend, 212
Lentil Bowl, 263–264
Lemon(s)
Citrus Boost, 241–242
Citrus Power Dressing, 260
Cranberry Green Tea Lemonade,
243–244
Lemon-Garlic Greens, 252–53
for liver detox, 75–76
Super-Detoxifying Green Tea
Lemonade, 243
Lentil Bowl, 263–264
Licorice root
for colon cleanse, 159–160
Colon Cleanse Herbal Tea,
246–247
Liquified petroleum gas, 27
Liver. *See also* Love Your Liver
Weekend
fatty, signs of, 70
functions of, 17, 67–68
Liver-boosting foods, top twelve,
73–77

Love Your Liver Weekend, 65–93
benefits, 65–66
conclusion of, 88
critical nutrients, 77–79
dietary suggestions, 71–77
exercises, 82–83
grocery list, 89–90
herbal liver boosters, 79–82
journal, 90–93
reasons for, 67–68
signs of stressed liver, 68–71
spa treatments, 83–86
weekend schedule, 86–88
worksheets, 89–93
Lymphatic system, 95–97. *See also*
Lymphomania Weekend
Lymphomania Weekend, 95–115
benefits of, 95
conclusion of, 111–112
critical nutrients, 102–103
dietary suggestions, 99–102
exercises, 105–106
grocery list, 112–113
herbal lymph system boosters,
103–105
journal, 113–115
reasons for detox, 95–98
signs of stressed lymphatic
system, 98, 111
spa treatments, 106–109
weekend schedule, 109–111
worksheets, 112–115

Magnesium, 129, 158
Maltose, 10
Massage Oil
fat-blasting, making your own, 224
Hormone-Balancing, 271–272
Massages
acupressure abdominal, 162–164
aromatherapy abdominal,
223–226
lymph-booster, 106–108

Meals, skipping, 56
Meals, small, 56, 207
Meat, 42, 180
Medications, 62–63
Meditation, 134–134
Melon
    Cantaloupe Ice, 241
    for skin rejuvenation, 181
    Watermelon Ice, 241
Menopause, 187
Menstrual periods, 187
Mercury, 43
Methyl, 23
Microbiome, 148–149
Milk, dairy, 41, 207
Milk, non-dairy, 55
Milk thistle, 80
Mint
    Cucumber Refresh, 240
    Kidney Herbal Tea, 246
    Love Your Liver Herbal Tea,
        244–45
    Lymphomania Herbal Tea, 245
    Mint-Cucumber Salad, 258
    Skin Rejuvenation Herbal Tea,
        247
Monosodium glutamate (MSG),
    17–20
Multivitamins/mineral supplements
    for colon cleanse, 157
    for detox weekends, 56–57
    for Fat Blast Weekend, 206, 213
    for kidney detox, 123, 127–128,
        130
    for liver cleansing, 77
    for lymph detox, 102
    for skin rejuvenation, 185–186
Mushroom, Portobello, Gravy,
    253–254
Myalgic encephalomyelitis (ME), 68

Neurotoxins, 47
Nuts
    for colon cleanse, 154

    for detox weekends, 54
    Herbes de Provence Cashew
        Cheese, 250–251
    for kidney detox, 124
    for liver detox, 72, 76
    for lymph detox, 100, 101
    Pumpkin Spice Drop Cookies,
        267–268
    for skin rejuvenation, 179,
        181, 183
    Thyroid-Boosting Chocolate
        Truffles, 268

Oats, gluten-free, 44–45
Obesity, 7, 9
Obesogens, 7
Oil, for massages. See Massage Oil
Oils. See also Flax seeds/flax
        seed oil
    Better Than Butter, 250
    canola, 22, 180
    coconut, 55
    cottonseed, 22
    for detox weekends, 55
    olive, 55, 180
    rancid, note about, 16–17
    for skin rejuvenation, 180
Olive flower remedy, 275
Olive oil, 55, 180
Omega 3 fatty acids, 42–43, 179,
        181, 182, 183, 185
Omega 6 fatty acids, 42
Onions, 76, 212
Organic foods, 46–48, 180
Osteoporosis, 41

Packaged foods, 38–39
Parkinson's disease, 48
Peanuts, 154
Pear Cranberry Juice, 242
Pepper(s)
    Roasted Red, Chickpea Mash, 263
    Veggie Scramble, 262–263
Perfume, 28

Perspiration, 176
Pesticides, 41, 43, 48
Petrolatum, 23
Petroleum distillate, 27
Phthalates, 7, 27
Pizza, 209
Plastic, toxins in, 6–7
Polychlorinated biphenyls (PCBs), 7–8
Potassium, 120, 130
Potato chips, 210
Poultry, for skin rejuvenation, 180
Prepared foods, 38–39
Probiotic powder
    Dairy-Free Yogurt, 248–249
    Herbes de Provence Cashew Cheese, 250–251
Probiotics, 128, 152, 157
Processed foods, 38–39
Propane, 27–28
Propyl, 23
Protease, 103
Protein
    avoiding sugar cravings with, 218
    for Fat Blast Weekend, 205–206
    in high-protein diets, 117, 119
    powder, MSG in, 18
Pumpkin, for skin rejuvenation, 182
Pumpkin Spice Drop Cookies, 267–268
Putyl, 23
PVP/VA copolymer, 23

Qigong, 58–59
Quinoa, about, 45
Quinoa Ginger Chili, 264

Rashes, 174–175
Rebounding, 105–106
Rescue Remedy, 276
Resveratrol, 214–215
Rice. See Brown rice; Wild rice

Saccharin, 14
Saffron, 217
Salad dressings
    Citrus Power Dressing, 260
    MSG in, 18
    Salade du Provence Dressing, 259–260
    suggestions for, 256
Salads
    adding fat-burning foods to, 256
    adding protein-rich toppings to, 256–257
    base ingredients for, 254
    Cucumber-Mint, 258
    for detox weekends, 51
    for Fat Blast Weekend, 205
    Heirloom Tomato and Basil, 257–258
    mix-ins for, 255
    toppings for, 255
    Weekend Wonder Detox Signature Salad, 258–259
Salmon, farmed, toxins in, 7
Salmon Parcels, 266
Salt, 46, 120
Salt body scrub, 191
SAMe (S-adenosylmethionine), 78, 79
Sanitizers, 27–28
Saturated fats, 16
Sauces, bottled, 18
Seaweed, 123–24, 126, 181–182
Seaweed skin treatments, 190
Seeds. See also Flax seeds/flax seed oil
    for colon cleanse, 154
    for detox weekends, 54
    for kidney detox, 124
    for liver detox, 72, 76
    for lymph detox, 100, 101
    for skin rejuvenation, 179, 182
Sideways leg lifts, 221–222

Skin. *See also* Skin Rejuvenation
    Weekend
  dry, brushing, 108–109
  function of, 174
  Skin Rejuvenation Herbal Tea,
    247
  Skin-Soothing Chapped Skin
    Ointment, 272
  Skin-Soothing Natural Body
    Lotion, 269–270
Skin Rejuvenation Weekend,
    173–199
  benefits of, 173–175
  conclusion of, 194
  critical nutrients, 183–186
  dietary suggestions, 178–183
  exercises, 187–188
  grocery list, 195–196
  herbal skin cleansers, 186–187
  journal, 196–199
  reasons for detox, 175–177
  signs of stressed-out skin,
    177–178
  spa treatments, 189–192
  weekend schedule, 192–194
  worksheets, 195–199
Snacks, 152, 207, 218
Soda, 40, 125, 211
Sodium, 120
Sodium laurel sulphates, 23
Soups
  Coconut Vegetable Soup, Thai,
    261–262
  Detox, Spicy, Rice-y, 260–261
  MSG in, 18
Soy foods, 21–22, 76, 212
Soy "meat" products, 18
Spa treatments
  acupressure abdominal massage,
    162–164
  acupressure for kidney detox and
    healing, 135–137
  acupressure for liver detox and
    healing, 83–85

aromatherapy abdominal
    massage, 223–226
aromatherapy compress, 85–86
aromatherapy skin softener bath,
    189–190
at-home thalassotherapy bath,
    190
dry skin brushing, 108–109
healthy kidney meditation,
    134–135
lymph-booster massage, 106–108
salt body scrub, 191
skin clarity facial, 191–192
Spice mixtures, 18
Spices, 55–56, 212, 213, 217
Spleen, 97
Splenda, 14–16
Sprouts, 52–53, 101
Squash
  for colon cleanse, 156
  and Garbanzo Bean Stew,
    Curried, 265
  Pumpkin Spice Drop Cookies,
    267–268
  for skin rejuvenation, 182
Squats, 222
Stearalkonium chloride, 24
Stevia, 39–40, 206
Stew, Curried Garbanzo Bean and
    Squash, 265
Strawberries, 182
Strength training, 219–223
Stress, 276
Stroke, 11
Sucralose, 14–16
Sugar
  cravings for, 217–218
  eliminating, in detox
    weekends, 39
  eliminating, in Fat Blast
    Weekend, 206
  eliminating, in kidney detox, 124
  genetically modified, 22
  health problems linked to, 9–10

Sunflower seeds, 182
Superoxide dismutase (SOD), 185
Supplements. *See* Multivitamins/
    mineral supplements
Sweat, 176
Sweeteners, 8–11. *See also* Artificial
    sweeteners
Sweet potatoes, for skin
    rejuvenation, 183
Sweet Potato Fries, 249

Tapioca, Chia Breakfast, 266–267
Taurine, 78
Tea. *See also* Green Tea
    Herbal, Colon Cleanse, 246–247
    Herbal, Kidney, 246
    Herbal, Love Your Liver,
        244–245
    Herbal, Lymphomania, 245
    Herbal, Skin Rejuvenation, 247
    Honey-Turmeric, 247
Thalassotherapy bath, 190
Thyroid-Boosting Chocolate
    Truffles, 268
Tofu
    Veggie Scramble, 262–263
Tomato(es)
    Heirloom, and Basil Salad,
        257–258
    Veggie Scramble, 262–263
Toothpaste, Natural, 273
Tortilla chips, 209
Trans fats, 16, 17, 211
Triceps extensions, 223
Truffles, Chocolate, Thyroid-
    Boosting, 268
Turmeric
    for Fat Blast Weekend, 212–213
    for kidney detox, 127
    for liver detox, 76–77, 81–82
    Turmeric-Honey Tea, 247

Urea, 119
Urination, 120–121

Vaccines, 18
Vegetable(s). *See also specific*
    vegetables
    buying, for juices, 239
    for colon cleanse, 151
    for detox weekends, 51–52
    juices, for detox weekends, 125,
        178–179, 204, 205
    for kidney detox, 123
    for liver detox, 71
    for lymph detox, 100
    Soup, Thai Coconut, 261–262
    Veggie Scramble, 262–263
Vitamins. *See also* Multivitamins/
    mineral supplements
    B-complex, 78–79, 157
    Vitamin A, 130, 184
    Vitamin C, 77–78, 102–103,
        128–129, 130
    Vitamin D3, 184
    Vitamin E, 130, 184

Walnut flower remedy, 275–276
Walnuts
    Pumpkin Spice Drop Cookies,
        267–268
    for skin rejuvenation, 183
Water
    avoiding sugar cravings
        with, 218
    body's need for, 48–50
    for detox weekends, 50
    for kidney detox, 124–125
    lack of, and kidneys, 119–120
    for skin rejuvenation, 178
Watermelon Ice, 241
Water supply, toxins in, 15–16,
    47
Weight gain
    from fruit, 40, 53
    from sluggish lymphatic
        system, 97
    top foods contributing to,
        208–211

Weight loss. *See also* Fat Blast
    Weekend
  top fat-blasting foods for, 211–213
Wheat products, 99
White walnut
  for colon cleanse, 160
  Colon Cleanse Herbal Tea,
    246–247
Wild indigo root, 105
Wild rice, 45
Wild rose flower remedy, 275

Worksheets, about, 60

Yellow dock
  for skin rejuvenation, 186
  Skin Rejuvenation Herbal Tea,
    247
Ylang ylang, about, 271
Yoga, 58, 132
Yogurt, Dairy-Free, 248–249

Zinc, 185